SOOTHE YOUR ACHES AND PAINS

THE NO NONSENSE LIBRARY

NO NONSENSE HEALTH GUIDES

Women's Health and Fitness
A Diet for Lifetime Health
A Guide to Exercise and Fitness Equipment
How to Tone and Trim Your Trouble Spots
Stretch for Health
Unstress Your Life
Calories, Carbohydrates and Sodium
Permanent Weight Loss
All about Vitamins and Minerals
Your Emotional Health and Well-Being
Reducing Cholesterol
Lower Your Blood Pressure
The Fiber Primer
Walk for Health

NO NONSENSE FINANCIAL GUIDES

NO NONSENSE REAL ESTATE GUIDES

NO NONSENSE LEGAL GUIDES

NO NONSENSE CAREER GUIDES

NO NONSENSE SUCCESS GUIDES

NO NONSENSE COOKING GUIDES

NO NONSENSE WINE GUIDES

NO NONSENSE PARENTING GUIDES

NO NONSENSE STUDENT GUIDES

NO NONSENSE AUTOMOTIVE GUIDES

NO NONSENSE PHOTOGRAPHY GUIDES

NO NONSENSE GARDENING GUIDES

NO NONSENSE HEALTH GUIDE®

SOOTHE YOUR ACHES AND PAINS

A Head-to-Toe Guide for Fast, Effective Relief

By the Editors of *PREVENTION* Magazine

Longmeadow Press

Notice

This book is intended as a reference volume only, not as a medical manual or guide to self-treatment. It is not intended as a substitute for the medical advice of physicians. The reader should regularly consult a physician in general, and particularly for any symptoms. If you suspect that you have a medical problem, we urge you to seek competent medical help. Keep in mind that exercise and nutritional needs vary from person to person, depending on age, sex, health status, and individual variations. The information here is intended to help you make informed decisions about your health, not as a substitute for any treatment that may have been prescribed by your doctor.

Library of Congress Cataloging-in-Publication Data

Soothe your aches and pains : a head-to-toe guide for fast, effective relief / by the editors of Prevention magazine.
      p.   cm. — (No nonsense health guide)
  ISBN 0–681–41019–1 paperback
  1. Pain—Popular works.   I. Prevention (Emmaus, Pa.) II. Series: No-nonsense health guide.
RB127.S66 1991
616' .0472—dc20
                                          90–25655
                                          CIP

Compiled and edited by Marcia Holman

Book design by Rodale Design Staff

Photographs by Angelo Caggiano, pp. 5, 86; Carl Doney, p. 42; Mitch Mandel, p. 49; Paul Pelak, p. 73; Rodale Stock Images, pp. 17, 22, 35, 61; Sally Shenk Ullman, p. 29.

Printed in the United States of America on acid-free paper ∞

0 9 8 7 6 5 4 3 2 1   paperback

Contents

Tapping Into Your Body's Natural Painkillers

Sooner or later, we all have our share of aches and pains. One survey revealed that three out of four adults experienced headaches in the course of a year. Half had muscle or joint pains, while four in ten adults experienced stomach pains. Nearly a third had dental pain. Another report tells us that the second most common cause for hospitalization in the United States is backache—right after childbirth!

It's easy to see why so many feel bullied by pain. Fortunately, you have a variety of effective painkilling weapons at your disposal.

One of the best, of course, is aspirin. Americans swallow an estimated 30 millon pounds of aspirin every year. And for good reason. Aspirin is an effective and inexpensive analgesic, or painkiller.

But taking aspirin—or any analgesic—in large amounts or for a long time can be harmful. Furthermore, painkillers mask the pain that acts as a warning signal, alerting you that something bad has happened to your body and that you need to pay heed. If you mask the signal and ignore the pain, you might develop even more serious problems.

Now here's the good news: Scientists have discovered that your body manufactures its own natural painkillers. What's more, there are a variety of physical and psychological ways you can encourage your body to produce them.

Much of this pain control research is based on the "gate control" theory of pain. According to this theory, when your body is injured in some way, substances called prostaglandins are released. These are chemical hormones that signal the nerve endings to send pain impulses through your body via distinct pathways. The pain impulses move through the tissues from nerve fiber to nerve fiber to the spinal cord and the "gate" before finally reaching the brain. And when the signal reaches the brain, you hurt.

One of the ways aspirin and similar pain-relieving drugs work is to interfere with prostaglandin production. But more natural means can also interrupt the pain signal on its way to the brain. A simple rubdown of an injured area, for example, can create a competing signal on the pathway to the brain. The two signals create a kind of traffic jam on the pathway and the gate closes. The pain signal can't get through, so you feel no pain.

Similarly, applying a cold compress to an inflamed joint is an excellent way to "close the gate" at the spinal pathway and inhibit painful information from reaching your brain.

Other nondrug practices, like gentle exercise and relaxation techniques, can help manage pain by stimulating production of endorphins, your body's pain-relieving hormones.

In *Soothe Your Aches and Pains,* you'll learn dozens of ways to switch on your body's natural painkillers so you can remain on your feet and feeling great. You'll discover, for example, how a hot shower can wash away tension headaches and how proper nutrition can tame those monster migraines. The do-it-on-the-spot pain relief techniques can help stop sinusitis, quell menstrual cramps, and ease muscular sprains.

Finally, you'll learn how you can adjust the way you stand, sit, and sleep to keep your muscles relaxed and your joints aligned, so pain can't take over your body in the future.

Turn Off Tension Headaches

You've got a headache so bad it feels as if your skull is being squeezed in a vise. What in the world could have caused this pain in your brain?

You hunched over your desk all day crunching numbers.

You drove 4 hours in bumper-to-bumper traffic to Vacation-land, U.S.A., with your kids whining, "Are we there yet?" every 10 minutes.

You fought with your spouse over who got butter in the jelly jar.

You watched three soaps, four game shows, a mini-series, and the colorized version of *The Maltese Falcon* on TV.

Like football or baseball, headaches are a national pastime. And headache relief is big business. A National Headache Foundation exists for headache researchers and headache sufferers. And the professional journal *Headache* is devoted exclusively to reporting on this problem.

"It's a very rare person indeed who has never experienced a

headache," says Seymour Solomon, M.D., director of the Headache Unit at Montefiore Medical Center in the Bronx.

Strain Causes Pain

Tension headache, also known as muscular contraction headache, is estimated to account for 90 percent of all headaches. In a tension headache, the muscles in your neck, jaw, face, and scalp contract or "tense up" for prolonged periods, causing steady, squeezing pain that makes you feel as if you're wearing a hat several sizes too small. Your neck and face muscles may feel stiff and tender.

Your muscles are most likely to cramp up and cause headache pain when you clench your teeth, frown, or squint for long periods or when you hold your body rigid or in an awkward position for too long. Emotional stress also can trigger a tension headache. A family crisis, dealing with deadlines at work, worrying about bills—you name it, when you're under stress, your body may react by constricting your head and neck muscles.

If you get tension headaches frequently, doctors say, it's likely that your body is biologically programmed to contract the muscles of your head and neck in a painful way and to keep them contracted—even when you're merely slightly stressed.

"What we're finding is that if you're headache prone, you may be more vulnerable to certain triggers, such as stress, for example, that can throw your serotonin out of balance and touch off a whole avalanche of symptoms in your body," says Joel Saper, M.D., director of the Michigan Headache and Neurological Institute in Ann Arbor. Serotonin's job is to help your brain direct many of your body's functions, including pain regulation, blood vessel dilation, and muscle contraction.

What this means is that something as ordinary as squabbling with your son about his curfew might sufficiently alter your serotonin level to make the muscles in your neck tense up. And tight neck muscles can create horrendous pain.

Go easy on aspirin.   For that once- or twice-a-month tension headache, over-the-counter painkillers like aspirin, acetaminophen (Tylenol), or ibuprofen (Nuprin) may work well. Certainly a lot of us think so—we spend more than $4 billion annually on these pills.

But if you tend to get tension headaches more frequently, popping aspirin like candy every day may not make a dent in your head pain. In fact, frequent aspirin use may make your headaches strike back with a vengeance. "Studies have shown that if you have a biological predisposition toward developing headaches, taking more than three to six aspirin a day could disrupt your serotonin level and could worsen your headaches," says Fred Sheftell, M.D., director of the New England Center for Headaches in Stamford, Connecticut.

So if you are prone to tension headaches, you may be better off using a nonpill approach for relief. Try one of these simple, safe methods to help you fight head pain and keep you on your feet next time a headache threatens to overshadow your day.

Relax Tight Muscles

Your best defense when your head feels like it's caught in a hammerlock may be to consciously relax the muscles that are causing the pain. Studies have shown that people who learn to relax their muscles can significantly reduce the number and intensity of their headaches. And there are lots of ways to achieve this relaxation. The following natural tension relievers could help you get out from under the grip of a headache:

Rub out pain.   "Having someone massage your shoulders and neck can be a great way to relax taut muscles," says Albert Elkind, M.D., director of the Elkind Headache Center in Mount Vernon, New York. "A massage stimulates muscle tissue, allows greater blood flow, and feels absolutely marvelous."

There are other reasons why a good rubdown can rub out head pain. When you're tense, your neck and head muscles contract, releasing prostaglandins. (As you recall from the Introduction, these are chemical hormones that signal the nerve endings to send pain impulses to the brain. Once the signal reaches the brain, you begin to hurt. Rubbing may snuff out your pain by keeping the pain signal from reaching the brain.)

What's more, rubbing erases pain by helping your body release endorphins—pain-relieving hormones that operate in the descending pathways from the brain.

A soothing self-massage.   If no one is around to massage your aches away, try this simple self-massage: Place both hands gently over your ears and hold for 30 seconds. Move your palms to the sides of your head and slide them in circles over both temples for another 30 seconds. Next, spread out your fingers, push your fingertips onto the top of your head, and rotate your scalp in as many directions as you can. Apply fairly strong pressure—you want to move the skin against the bone. Move your fingertips over your scalp repeating this massage several times until you've worked your entire head.

Press here for relief.   Pressing certain specific points on your body seems to make the body produce more endorphins. That's the idea behind acupuncture, the Chinese tradition of inserting superfine needles at prescribed sites on the body. Acupuncture apparently excites the endorphin systems. Acu*pressure* supposedly works the same way, except you stimulate the nerves with your thumbs or fingers instead of needles. Two key points for reducing head pain with acupressure are the web between the forefinger and thumb (squeeze there until you feel pain), and under the bony ridges at the back of the neck.

To apply pressure at the back of your neck, feel the back of your head about level with the earlobe, and find two bumps—one on each side of the midline. Lower your fingers about an inch until you are under the bumps. Rock your head slightly back until you feel the neck muscles relax. Bring your elbows forward so that you can massage those muscles with your fingertips.

Turn on the tap.   Stand under a hot shower and aim the stream of water at the back of your neck. What happens when you do this, says Glen Solomon, M.D., of the Headache Section of the Cleveland Clinic, is that you stimulate blood flow that flushes away prostaglandins. Or use a hot water bottle as a pillow. Place it at the back of your neck and sit back in your easy chair—ahh, feel your neck muscles slowly unwind and your headache disappear.

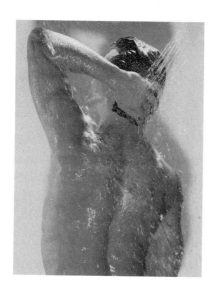

Next time a tension headache strikes, your defense may be as near as your hot-water tap. Aim the shower stream on your neck muscles. The warm water helps unkink tight muscles and stimulates the blood flow—ahh—headache pain is washed away!

Pay Attention to Posture

One of the best ways to relieve muscular tension anywhere, anytime, is to do some simple postural adjustments, known as retraction exercises. "Much of the pain in tension headaches arises from overstretching your neck muscles and thrusting your head forward like a turtle," explains Joanne Griffin, registered physical therapist at the Headache Clinic at Greenwich Hospital in Connecticut. "You can often relieve pain by drawing back your shoulders and gently aligning your head at the top of your spine where it belongs." The easiest way to achieve this correct, pain-free posture is to keep your eyes forward and then simply slide your head back, making a double chin.

Use a well-placed pillow.   Another way to relieve a headache is to sit in a chair with a small rolled-up towel placed in the hollow of your back, near your belt line. A well-placed pillow will gently force your lower back into the correct curvature, put your shoulders and head back, and allow you to sit with less muscle strain. "Just making this simple adjustment at the first hint of a headache can keep it from becoming a full-blown assault,"says Griffin.

Don't be a stomach sleeper.   Sleeping on your stomach can put too much pressure on the side of your jaw and neck, causing a headache.

Also, toss out those rock-hard or feather-soft pillows—they tense up your neck muscles. Look for cervical pillows—tube-shaped pillows that give your neck the support without tensing the muscles. A folded towel placed under your neck might work, too.

Do the body scan.   Throughout the day, check yourself for signs that you are tensing up and inviting headache—clenched teeth, clenched fists, hunched shoulders.

Notice any postural habits that may be sparking your muscle contraction headaches. One woman found, for example, that her headaches came on when she was chopping vegetables for a dinner party or sewing draperies. She discovered that the intense concentration involved in these activities made her clench her teeth for so long that her head hurt.

Be aware of how you hold your head while at work or driving or reading. Make sure you're not holding your body in one position for too long. Avoid postures that twist your neck or pull your head forward like a turtle. Don't slump with your chin on your chest when watching TV or reading. And don't chew gum: The repetitive chewing motion can tighten muscles and bring on a tension headache.

Practice tension prevention.   To prevent tension buildup, periodically shift your position, shake out your arms, and slowly bend your head from side to side and from back to front.

Move to Unkink Muscles

Halting a really tough tension headache once it's taken hold may take a little more effort than shifting positions. Sometimes you have to make a conscious effort to loosen up muscles so that stiffness—and pain—does not set in.

Head rolls help.   First, get into your proper posture—eyes straight, chin pulled back. Next, take several slow, deep breaths. Then begin to slowly rotate your head in circles, first to the left and then to the right. Next, bend one ear toward your shoulder. Repeat with the opposite ear. Finally, rotate each shoulder in forward circles a few times and then in backward circles. This gentle stretching can loosen up even the tightest muscles.

On-the-spot stretch.   Here's a quick way to unkink muscles if you're stuck in traffic. Grasp the top of the steering wheel with both hands, making sure your forearms are also resting on the wheel. Scoot your backside against the back of the seat. Now hunch your upper body forward and arch like a frightened cat. Hold for a few seconds and repeat. You may look a bit strange to the guy in the next lane, but you'll feel great.

Move, move, move.   The first chance you can get to move your entire body, do so. On a long-distance drive, stop for a stroll at the nearest highway rest area, for instance. Many people find that more vigorous movement, like a brisk walk or even running, is a great way to melt stiffness and chase away a tension headache. "It's possible that exercise may help your body produce endorphins, your body's natural painkilling hormones," says Dr. Elkind.

Regular exercise is also a great way to *prevent* tension headaches. The reason? It helps discharge stress.

Find Peace and Relaxation

When you learn how to release the tension from your muscles, you can release the pain from your head. There are a variety of ways that will help you release muscular tension, defuse stress and eliminate headaches so that you can enjoy a healthy, active life.

Breathe deeply.   Deep breathing is a great tension reliever. "You're doing it right," Dr. Sheftell says, "if your stomach is moving more than your chest."

You might also try putting a pencil between your teeth without biting. You have to relax to do this.

Try progressive relaxation and imagery.   Find a quiet space. Sit in a comfortable chair, or lie on the floor, and breathe deeply and regularly. Now tense and then relax each muscle group in your body, starting with your feet and working up your body to the top of your head and ending with your arms and hands.

Now imagine the tension flowing out of your body through your fingertips. At the same time, imagine yourself in your favorite surroundings, whether on a tropical beach, on a ski slope, or before a glowing fireplace.

For shortcut imagery that produces the same effect, try this: "Imagine the muscle fibers in your neck and head to be all scrunched up," says Dr. Sheftell. "Then begin to *smooth* them out in your mind."

Learn biofeedback.   Studies have shown that people who use biofeedback machines to help them relax are able to nip tension-headache pain in the bud. After about four weeks of training, patients often learn to relax quickly at the first sign of a headache by sitting quietly and repeating the calming phrases.

Getting hooked up to a biofeedback machine is a simple procedure. Electrodes placed over your scalp and neck muscles are wired to a machine that produces one kind of audible tone that indicates when your muscles are being tensed and another tone when muscles are relaxed. Your goal is to learn to change the tone to the relaxed pitch by consciously relaxing your muscles and repeating relaxing phrases.

Ask your doctor about where to go to learn biofeedback therapy.

Taming Monster Migraines

Migraines have been called the Sherman tank of headaches— the heavyweight headaches that two aspirin can't touch. Unlike tension headaches, migraines produce a sharp, throbbing pain, usually on one side of the head. Many people who feel pain in their foreheads, temples, or around their eyes assume they have sinus problems but in fact have migraines. These headaches hit you hard, and the pain is persistent, pounding, punishing. All you want to do is crawl into a dark hole and wait until the pain passes.

If you get migraines, you're not alone. An estimated 12 million sufferers are pummeled by the pain of migraines.

One reason you feel such intense pain when you get a migraine is that your blood vessels swell up and press on the nerve endings in your head, releasing substances that cause intense head pain. Your pain may last several hours to several days, and you may experience nausea, vomiting, dizziness, tender skin, or a sensitivity to light.

Migraines usually give some kind of warning before the actual pain strikes. You may crave sweets, become depressed or tired, or even feel unusually exhilarated or hyperactive. In some cases, an arm or leg may go numb or you may see flashing lights before your eyes.

Migraines Remain a Mystery

The exact cause for this punishing ailment has remained a mystery despite the fact that migraines have afflicted millions of people throughout history, including some of the greatest minds— Julius Ceasar, Thomas Jefferson, Frederic Chopin, and Virginia Woolf, to name a few.

"Perhaps no other condition of such magnitude has been surrounded by more myth and misinformation or has been more misunderstood than migraine headaches," says Joel Saper, M.D., director of the Michigan Headache and Neurological Institute in Ann Arbor.

Back in the Middle Ages, for example, headaches were believed to be the work of evil spirits. That belief led many an unfortunate sufferer to submit to having a hole drilled in the skull so that the alleged demons could escape.

Fortunately, scientists have gotten closer to discovering the true causes for headaches and are coming up with a variety of methods for exorcising one of humanity's most cruel forms of pain—methods that are gentle, fast acting, and effective even for the most hellish headaches.

Blame Your Pain on Your Genes

While you can no longer point to the devil as the cause of your headaches, there may be good reason to blame a family disposition.

"Like chronic tension headaches, chronic migraine headaches appear to be an inherited, biological disease," says Dr. Saper. "If you're prone to migraine headaches, chances are you have a mother, aunt, or someone else in the family who suffers or *had* suffered frequent head pain."

Dr. Saper explains that if you get more than an occasional migraine, you probably have an inherited tendency for the brain chemical serotonin to fluctuate. Serotonin, you may recall from chapter 1, is the neurotransmitter responsible for pain regulation, blood vessel dilation, and muscle contraction. In addition, serotonin is also in charge of controlling your appetite, your sleep center, your senses, even your emotions.

What all this means is that if something throws your serotonin level out of balance, you may not only get a whopping head pain, you may also experience a variety of other unpleasant symptoms commonly associated with migraines.

The Major Migraine Triggers

If you are ambushed by migraines frequently, you may be susceptible to specific triggers—such as certain foods, hormones, or stress—that can disrupt your serotonin level and set off a cascade of events in your body. Drinking a glass of wine, for example, might alter your serotonin level sufficiently to make the blood vessels in your head dilate. And dilated blood vessels can press on your nerve endings and give you a nightmare of a headache. At the same time, an altered serotonin level could cause your appetite or moods to go haywire. You may feel nauseous, fatigued, or irritable.

A host of other triggers can light the migraine fuse. The flickering glare of the TV, a sunny day, skipping lunch, taking a noonday snooze, even a change in weather can trigger a major headache.

A delayed stress reaction.   As with tension headaches, stress can trigger a migraine. Yet for many migraine victims, the pain doesn't set in until after the emotionally distressing event has passed. For example, your migraine may wait in the wings all during the stressful week before your vacation but hit you full force the first chance you get to relax. The reason? During the stressful period, your blood vessels overly constrict. Then, when you relax, your blood vessels "let down," that is, they dilate, and voilà— you get a vacation-spoiling migraine.

A matter of hormones.   One of the biggest headache provokers for women is too little or too much of the hormone estrogen. Migraines strike women three times more often than men and, experts say, more than half of women's migraines are related to changes in the estrogen level.

Many women, in fact, remain headache-free all month until their period begins. During the first few days of menstruation, estrogen levels fluctuate, and in some women, this estrogen fluctuation may alter the serotonin level sufficiently to trigger a horrendous headache.

How to Shrink Swollen Vessels

When you're in the throes of a migraine, all you may want to do is, as one sufferer put it, ''crawl in a dark hole and shut out the world.'' The reason you crave isolation is that during a migraine attack, you become supersensitive to outside stimuli—even looking at the lighted numbers of a digital clock could be excruciating.

Fortunately, you can relieve these headaches even when you *can't* go home and pull up the covers. The key to heading off migraines is to quickly shrink swollen blood vessels in your head.

Drink one cup of coffee.   One way to reduce swollen vessels is to have a cup of coffee or a cola. These beverages contain caffeine, and caffeine constricts the blood vessels—that's why it's included in most pain medications. But don't go overboard. More than two mugs of coffee or cans of cola could *over*constrict your blood vessels, making them react later by overdilating. The result is a whopping head pain.

Put your vessels on ice.   Placing something cold against your brow is another way to constrict swollen vessels. You might try holding a cold washcloth, or better yet a cold gel pack, against your forehead for a half hour or so. In one study, more than half of the migraine sufferers got immediate relief after applying a cold pack.

You can also foil a migraine by resting your neck on a cold

pack. Design your own special cervical pillow. Roll up ice cubes in a thin towel and place the roll at the bottom of your pillow case. Your blood vessels will shrink and you'll be able to drift off to dreamland.

Seek a cool room.   Since heat prompts blood vessels to dilate, just sitting quietly in an air-conditioned room or a shady, wooded spot can be enough to abort a migraine.

Touch your temples.   ''When you press on or near the pain spot, you block the pain sensation with the pressure sensation,'' says Albert Elkind, M.D., director of the Elkind Headache Center in Mount Vernon, New York. So find those little indentations midway between the corners of your eyes and the tops of your ears. Now, press the flat part of your thumbs firmly on these spots for several seconds. That could be enough to squelch a migraine.

Focus on a hand-warming image.   As odd as this technique may sound, experts say that imagining your hands are warm can actually arrest a migraine attack. Studies have shown that people who have learned to mentally warm their hands have fewer migraines, although doctors are unsure why. ''Supposedly, when when you imagine your hands getting warmer, you draw blood from your head, shrink your blood vessels, and thereby reduce migraine symptoms,'' Dr. Elkind explains.

Plug into biofeedback.   Just as a biofeedback machine can help muscles relax and stave off a tension headache, such a machine can help you get the knack of hand warming so you can stamp out a migraine. Some machines involve attaching thermometer-like sensors that detect the skin temperature of your hands. When you start to think about your hands getting warmer, the machine ''feeds back'' your progress by allowing you to see your skin temperature rise on the thermometer. In other words, a biofeedback machine teaches you what it feels like to make your hands warmer so that you'll be able to reproduce the feeling without the machine. Your doctor can tell you where to find biofeedback therapy.

How to Head off Headaches

Are you doomed to migraine pain just because you inherited the headache gene? Definitely not, says Dr. Saper. "Headaches don't have to be a way of life for you. Just because you have inherited a tendency to develop headaches does not mean that you are destined to be a headache victim any more than inheriting high blood pressure means you will automatically have a heart attack."

There are a host of measures you can take to short-circuit your head pain and reduce your risk of having a severe headache attack in the future. You can keep head pain permanently at bay by learning what provokes your headaches and modifying your posture, your diet, and your responses to stress.

Keep a headache diary.   The key to outwitting your headaches is to get to know your enemy.

To find out what your particular headache triggers might be, keep a diary for a few months. Note the frequency and severity of your headaches, and whether you feel a dull, all-over ache or a throbbing, localized pain or both symptoms. Make a note of what happened before the headache occurred—including what you were doing, eating, feeling, and even what the weather was like.

Your diary will help you track the pattern of attacks and see if there are any recurring triggers. Once you discover what may be causing your headaches, you can take steps to modify these triggers.

Activities to avoid.   Bright lights, disturbed body rhythms (like sleeping late), or certain odors can all upset the balance of serotonin in your body and set off a horrendous head pain. Here are five precautions to take if you are migraine prone:

Protect your eyes. Bright light—be it from the sun, fluorescent lighting, television, or a video display terminal (VDT)—can lead to squinting, eyestrain, and finally a headache. Sunglasses are a good idea if you're going to be outside. If you're working inside, take some rest breaks from the VDT screen and also wear some type of tinted glasses.

Don't nap. Too much sleep, even a nap, can cause a rapid drop in blood sugar, cause blood vessel dilation, and bring on a migraine. So get up at the same time, all the time—even on weekends and vacations. And don't burn the midnight oil, either. Fatigue also can trigger migraines.

Say "no de cologne." Strong perfume (and scented products) can set off a migraine.

Don't smoke and drive. Smoking releases carbon monoxide. And whenever carbon monoxide shows up, people get headaches. Smoking with the car windows down when you're driving in heavy traffic gives you a double dip of carbon monoxide. This gas appears to adversely affect brain blood flow, according to Dr. Saper. Also, nicotine—another bad guy—gets into your system. It actually interferes with some of the drugs used to control migraines, such as beta-blockers. As a result, doctors often have to increase the dosage, which can increase the chance of side effects.

Don't skip meals. Going more than five hours without food could throw off your serotonin level, causing your blood vessels to swell up. A midafternoon snack, for example, can head off late-in-the-day pain, even if all you eat is a couple of crackers or a piece of fruit.

Modify Your Menu

Your menu could be a potential mine field of migraine triggers. In fact, experts implicate food in about 25 percent of migraine headaches.

Certain foods, once absorbed into the bloodstream, act to either constrict or dilate blood vessels in the head, resulting in headaches. But not everybody is affected by each food in the same way. Here's how to find out if foods are causing your pain:

Track down and eliminate suspects.   The most effective way to test for a food sensitivity is to make a note of when your headaches occur and recall what foods you ate prior to the headache. Since most of these diet offenders act swiftly, often producing symptoms within 45 mintues of being consumed, it's not too difficult to tell what meal triggered the problem.

If your headaches seem to occur soon after eating any one or more of these foods, it would be wise to avoid them for a month or so. You may notice that you can lessen your headache pain considerably. Researchers found that when headache sufferers eliminated foods containing common additives and preservatives, for example, they had only half as many headaches as usual.

You might also find that if you make the following modifications in your menu, your migraines disappear:

Go easy on the jolt of java.   Caffeine in moderation, as already mentioned, may relieve headaches in some people by narrowing already widened vessels, but it also has a rebound effect when overused. On the other hand, if you cut back on caffeine suddenly, you may get withdrawal symptoms. The blood vessels, normally used to a slight narrowing from caffeine, swell and begin to pound, leaving you in pain. So gradually cut caffeine intake to about a cup or two a day.

Tame your sweet tooth.   Having a couple of glazed doughnuts for breakfast may make your blood sugar level soar and then drop rapidly. And a rapid dip in blood sugar could set off a headache. So go easy on the sweets.

Steer clear of beer and wine.   Alcohol literally goes to your head—it can trigger the pain mechanism, dilate the blood vessels, and give you a monstrous migraine. For some people, sipping red wine can mean the end of the celebration. Red wine (and brandy, as well) contains tyramine, an amino acid which can influence serotonin and bring on a headache. If you do drink, stick to white wine, or better yet, have a spritzer without the spirits.

Don't say cheese.   As long as you're passing up the wine, you might also steer clear of the cheese tray and the raisin-and-nut dish as well. These foods also contain tyramine, and if you are sensitive, nibbling on these foods could trigger a headache and signal the end of the party for you. Other tyramine-containing foods include pork, sour cream, yogurt, citrus fruits (particularly oranges), and vegetables (particularly spinach and onions).

Say no to chocolate.   Hey, it's fattening anyway. It also contains tyramine. The good news is that many young people outgrow this chemical reaction—the body appears to build up a tolerance.

Pass up the deli food.   Be on the lookout for headaches that come on after you sample meats from the deli tray. Pastrami, corned beef, and ham, as well as hot dogs and luncheon meats, are cured with nitrites, a preservative that can dilate blood vessels and bring on a major migraine.

Look out for MSG.   If you love eating Chinese food but notice that the moo goo gai pan gives you a dragon-sized head pain, the culprit may be MSG. Monosodium glutamate, a flavor enhancer used in Chinese cuisine and many processed foods, can bring on a throbbing pain within a half hour in certain individuals who have difficulty metabolizing this substance. So read labels carefully and ask the chef to hold the MSG.

Eat ice cream slowly.   You can probably remember more than one occasion when you ate a big bite of ice cream and seconds later felt an intense rush of pain to your head. Eat ice cream slowly, Dr. Saper advises, ''so that your palate will cool gradually instead of receiving a shock of cold.''

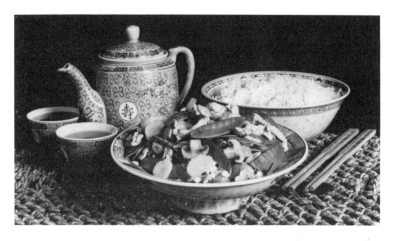

Does your head feel as if it's been hit with a gong not long after you eat Chinese food? If so, suspect the monosodium glutamate (MSG). This vessel-dilating additive often used in Chinese dishes can trigger a migraine headache, especially if you eat it on an empty stomach. Play it safe. Order your meal minus the MSG and start off with fresh fruit that is likely to be MSG-free.

CHAPTER
THREE

The Best Ways to Beat Sinusitis

You wake up at dawn with pounding pain in your head—everywhere, it seems: Your eyes, your nose, your forehead, even your teeth hurt. Your nose is so stuffed up you'd need RotoRooter to unplug it, and thick, vile-tasting fluid keeps dripping down the back of your throat.

A cold turned killer? Close. What you've probably got is sinusitis—inflammation and usually infection of one or more of the eight small cavities within your head called the paranasal sinuses that produces pressure, pain, and gobs of yellow or green mucus. Anywhere from 30 to 50 million Americans suffer this problem, making sinusitis one of the five most common health complaints in the country.

"Sinusitis is simply an inflammation of the membranes lining the sinuses that can interfere with normal drainage," says J. R. B. Hutchinson, M.D., president of the American Academy of Otolaryngic Allergy.

Sound simple? That's because it is. The big question: Why

does such a simple condition cause so many problems?

The mucus produced in our sinuses normally flushes out germs and debris that might otherwise cause infection. When the sinuses become inflamed, drainage stops. When drainage is interrupted for any reason, problems can develop. Sometimes the structure of the nose itself is partly to blame.

"All the sinuses drain into one small nasal area with an outlet about the size of the open tip of a ballpoint pen," explains Richard Mabry, M.D., clinical professor of otolaryngology at the University of Texas Southwestern Medical Center in Dallas. "The nose is very easily plugged up, and when that happens, the trapped fluid becomes the perfect medium for bacterial growth, usually leading to infection."

The congestion of severe sinusitis creates pressure around the eyes and forehead as well as pain in and around the sinuses. Sinusitis can also be accompanied by mild fever and thick discharge from the nose and down the back of the throat—the infamous postnasal drip.

Liquid Protection

Produced in your nose and sinuses, mucus contains substances that attack and kill marauding bacteria that happen to land in your respiratory tract.

In a typical day, your body produces about a quart of this key fluid, most of which you swallow without noticing. But when sinusitis hits, the mucus thickens. "People may think they are producing more mucus than usual, but what changes is not so much the volume as its thickness," says Dr. Hutchinson.

Postnasal drip can actually be a good sign: It means your sinuses are draining, which is important in defeating the infection. It can also be useful in diagnosing sinusitis. If you've got an allergy or just a cold, the mucus will usually be relatively clear and free-flowing. If you've got sinusitis from a bacterial infection, the discharge will change from clear and runny to a thicker consistency that looks more yellow or greenish.

How do you tell a bad cold from sinusitis? The key distinction is the course of the infection, and that takes some time to develop.

"A cold normally starts to get better after about 72 hours," explains Dr. Mabry. "It may drag on for a week, but most of us notice improvement starting around the third day. Sinusitis is the exact opposite: It gets worse after two or three days and continues to worsen."

The message here: If your cold gets worse after three days, or you notice a key symptom of sinusitis—increased pain, fever, or a change in nasal discharge—see your doctor immediately.

The Cause of Your Misery

The causes of sinusitis are just as varied as its symptoms, since essentially anything that produces inflammation in the nose can generate sinusitis. But most cases are caused by one of the three following factors.

Allergies.   Allergic symptoms can very closely mimic sinusitis: Your nose is so stuffed up you can't breathe. But with allergies, even when your nose starts running, your sinuses may still drain. Problems begin when allergic congestion blocks drainage from the sinus cavities, actually causing sinusitis.

"The medical history of people who repeatedly come down with sinusitis may not show any clues that an allergy is involved. And often you can't find any indication of a structural abnormality. I find that cases like this are strong indicators to look for an underlying allergy," Dr. Hutchinson says.

Environmental irritants.   Pollution is a tremendously important factor in sinusitis. Common pollutants include ozone, associated with automobile and industrial exhausts, and that nefarious nemesis, tobacco smoke.

"Tobacco is probably the worst offender," says Lee E. Smith, M.D., assistant clinical professor, Department of Otolaryngology—Head and Neck Surgery at the University of West Virginia. "Hot smoke loaded with tar—it's hard to imagine a worse combination." But again, anything that irritates the nose, be it fumes from the local paint factory or your neighbor's backyard barbecue, can bring on sinusitis.

Climate and geography play major roles in environmental

sinusitis. The wetter the climate in your part of the country, the more likely you are to encounter the pollens and other foliage-linked irritants that can cause sinusitis. Valleys can act as natural traps for pollutants and pollens, but if you live by the ocean, your risk is lower: The endless breezes sweep air clean.

"I hardly ever saw a case of sinusitis when I worked at Stanford University in California," Dr. Smith says. "I was absolutely astounded at how many I encountered when I moved to West Virginia, and I think climate and geography are chiefly responsible. Molds, pollens, and pollutants seem to affect people more severely here."

Structural abnormalities.   This generally means just one thing—a deviated septum, usually diagnosed either through visual examination of the nose or by X-ray. The septum is the cartilage-and-bone wall that separates the two air passages in your nose. Calling it deviated simply means it's crooked. When the septum is crooked, one of the air passages is narrower than the other, and that can lead to blockages.

"This condition is very common," says Dr. Hutchinson. "It's usually the result of a trauma—a fist fight, an automobile accident, or a sports injury, such as a catcher missing the ball and getting hit in the face. What patients notice most is that they have trouble breathing through one nostril or that one side of the nose gets congested whenever they lie down. This is one of the most common causes of chronic sinusitis, since the path of drainage is blocked."

Unclogging Your Head

Here's what the doctors suggest you do to unstuff your sinuses, reduce pain and pressure, and get the air flowing freely.

Sniff some steam.   "Humidity is the key to keeping the cilia working, the mucus flowing, and the sinuses drained," says Stanley N. Farb, M.D., chief of otolaryngology at Montgomery and Sacred Heart Hospitals, Norristown, Pennsylvania. Twice a day, stand in a shower hot enough to fog up the mirror. Or lean over a pan full of steaming water with a towel draped over your

Here's a quick way to unclog your stuffy sinuses: Get a steaming hot mug of coffee, tea, or soup. Cup your hands over the top of the mug, hold the mug up to your face, and sniff. The steamy vapors can help dissolve pain in seconds.

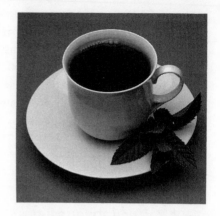

head, creating a steam tent. Inhale the vapors as they waft up toward your nostrils.

Moisturize the air.   Running a cold-mist machine in your bedroom will keep your nasal and sinus passages from drying out, says Bruce Jafek, M.D., chairman of otolaryngology/head and neck surgery at the University of Colorado School of Medicine. Just make sure you clean it once a week so fungus can't set up shop.

Try a nasal bath.   To flush out stale nasal secretions, use a commercial saline product or mix 1 teaspoon of table salt with 2 cups of warm water and a pinch of baking soda. Pour it into a shot glass, tilt your head back, close one nostril with your thumb, and sniff the solution with the open nostril. Then blow your nose gently. Repeat on the other side.

Drink fluids frequently.   Drinking extra liquids—both hot and cold—throughout the day thins out the mucus and keeps it flowing. Sipping hot teas made with herbs such as fenugreek, fennel, anise, or sage may help move mucus even more.

Rub for relief.   Rubbing your sore sinuses brings a fresh blood supply—and soothing relief—to the area. With one hand over each eye, rub steadily on the ridges of bone located just above and below your eyes. Then go after those sinuses hiding directly below your eyes and just above your teeth. Use your fingertips, thumbs, knuckles—whatever it takes to stop the pain.

Apply a warm washcloth.   Applying moist heat over tender sinuses is an easy way to wash away sinus pain. Apply a warm washcloth over your eyes and cheekbones and leave it there until you feel the pain subside. It may only take a few minutes.

Blow one nostril at a time.   This will help prevent pressure buildup in the ears, which can send bacteria further back into the sinus passages.

Walk to clear your head.   Exercise may bring blessed relief because it releases adrenaline, which constricts the blood vessels, thereby possibly reducing swelling in the sinuses.

Choose the right drug to "unstuff your doze."   The best over-the-counter medication to dry up sinuses is a single-action tablet that contains only decongestants, such as Sudafed. Decongestants constrict the blood vessels, put air through the nose, and alleviate pressure.

You should avoid products containing antihistamines if you are stuffed up from an infection. Antihistamines reduce swelling and let you breathe a little easier, but they also dry up the nose and thicken the mucus—exactly the opposite of what you want to do. Drainage is what you want, not dryness.

Use nasal sprays sparingly.   Nose drops are fine to use in a pinch, but frequent use could actually prolong the condition or even make it worse, warns Terence M. Davidson, M.D., director of the Nasal Dysfunction Clinic at the University of California Medical Center in San Diego. It's what specialists call "the rebound effect."

"What happens is that, initially, the sprays shrink your nasal linings," explains Dr. Davidson. "But then the mucosa reacts by swelling even more than before, creating a vicious cycle of use. It can take weeks for the swelling to finally subside after you stop using the sprays."

Know when to seek treatment.   If, after trying these treatments for three days, there is no improvement, see your doctor. The treatment is usually antibiotics, sometimes steroids, or at worst, surgery. Failing to treat sinusitis could lead to serious multiple-bacteria infections and much more serious disorders.

Sure-Fire Ways to Relieve TMJ

Lynn heard a cracking sound whenever she moved her mouth—and it wasn't because she was eating peanut brittle. That disturbing sound was Lynn's first clue that she had TMJ problems. The temporomandibular joints, or TMJs, connect the lower jaw to the skull; and when they act up, the symptoms can be disconcerting, not to mention painful.

After the cracking continued for a while, the 29-year-old Pennsylvania graphic artist recalls having difficulty opening her mouth wide. That was her second sign of trouble.

Finally, something happened to make it all too obvious that Lynn's jaw joints were not behaving as good joints should: she yawned, and—to her astonishment—her mouth locked open. Only by shoving her jaw with her hand could she get it to close. After this happened, Lynn decided it was time to seek medical attention.

She did, and now her TMJ problems are gone.

The TMJ Triggers

What caused Lynn's TMJ disorder in the first place? No one can say for sure, but it might have been related to the car accident she was in several years back.

Auto injuries or blows to the face and head are among the most common causes of TMJ problems, says Joseph L. Konzelman, D.D.S., clinical director of oral health research at the Walter Reed Army Medical Center in Washington, D.C., and past president of the American Academy of Oral Medicine.

Other causes of TMJ problems may include excessive teeth clenching or an irregular bite that doesn't allow the jaw to open and close evenly.

It's often hard to pinpoint the exact cause. "There are a large number of disorders that affect the TMJs, just as there are a lot of disorders that affect all joints in the body," says Dr. Konzelman. The problems can be related to muscles, ligaments, bones, cartilage, or a combination of these, he says.

Furthermore, the symptoms vary considerably. A locked jaw, such as Lynn experienced, is rare. More commonly, the prime giveaways of TMJ problems are facial pain and restricted jaw movement. You might also experience headache; toothache; aching neck, shoulders, or back; or a clicking or popping noise when opening or closing your jaw.

If you have any of these signs, check with an expert. "Professional diagnosis is the key to determining what is wrong and what to do about it. Call your family dentist and ask if he can help you or refer you to someone who can," says Dr. Konzelman. TMJ disorders tend to fall more under the practice of dentistry than under general medicine, he explains.

After you get a professional evaluation, what next? That depends on the nature of your specific problem, but there are a number of things that experts have found often give relief.

Posture Plays a Major Role

Dealing with the pain and discomfort of TMJ syndrome often starts with changing behavior that may be causing, or at least contributing to, your condition.

Six Self-Tests for TMJ Trouble

Can you give yourself a simple self-examination to tell if you've got TMJ problems? Unfortunately, an exact diagnosis of this complicated disorder is sometimes difficult even for medical professionals. You can, however, get an idea of whether or not you *may* have TMJ by testing yourself in the following ways.

1. Place the first two fingertips of each hand directly in front of each ear. The TMJs are directly underneath your fingers, and you should be able to feel their movement as you open and close your mouth. If even the light pressure of your fingertips causes pain on one or both sides, joint inflammation is a possibility.

2. Hold your hands on the sides of your face, so the fingertips are pointing toward your ears. Place all four fingers against the lower jaw on each side, with the index finger near the angle of the jaw. As you open and close your mouth you can feel the thick masseter muscles that extend diagonally from the angle to the cheekbone. Is there any pain?

3. Press your fingers lightly against your temples

Extending the neck while working at a desk or a computer is a fairly common cause of TMJ woes, says Dr. Konzelman. A chair with elbow supports should help you to keep your back straight, which will prevent you from leaning over the desk and holding your neck out. You may also find that a support pillow behind your lower back can make a difference.

If you work at a desk, check your body position throughout the day; make sure you—and especially your chin—are not leaning over the desk. As a general guideline for sitting or standing, your cheekbone shouldn't extend past your collarbone, and your ears should not be too far in front of your shoulders, he says.

Sitting for long periods in a seat where you can't cross your above and in front of your ears. Open and close your mouth. If you feel pain, one or both of the fan-shaped temporalis muscles may be fatigued and sore.

4. This resistance test will help you spot possible fatigue and soreness of the less-accessible muscles in the jaws: With the mouth partly open, press three fingers against the biting surfaces of the lower front teeth firmly but not hard. Try to close the jaw against this resistance. If this causes discomfort, see your dentist for a professional diagnosis.

5. With the jaw closed, press a fist against your chin and open against the resistance. Here again, any discomfort is a sign of trouble and should be checked out.

6. For your last test, press against each side of the lower jaw in turn and move it sideways against resistance. Is there any discomfort or pain? If so, you should seek an expert's advice.

legs, such as on an airplane or bus, may also put your body into the kind of awkward position that spells trouble for your TMJs. What's the answer? "If you can't cross your legs, at least elevate one buttock with a small magazine," says Dr. Konzelman. This can relieve some of the pressure.

Adopting an Anti-TMJ Lifestyle

You may not know it, but how you eat, sleep, even the clothes you wear may be giving you a pain in the jaws.

Take those chewy bagels you love to eat while reading the Sunday paper, for instance. Chomping on tough foods, like day-old bagels and raw carrots, can strain the jaw muscles. You may find that a softer diet will ease your pain. Substitute cooked vegetables and fruits for raw foods and eat pasta or casseroles in place of chewy steaks. Avoid chewing gum.

Now consider how you like to read your newspaper. Do you make a habit of reading while lying on your back with your head propped up at a sharp angle? That's another bad habit to break if you want to ease the pain in your jaws. Overcoming TMJ is very much a matter of what you *don't* do, claims Andrew S. Kaplan, D.M.D., an assistant clinical professor of dentistry at Mount Sinai School of Medicine of the City University of New York and author of *The TMJ Book*. If any of the following habits apply to you—pay attention! These tips may be of help to you.

Don't:
- Lie on your stomach with your head twisted to one side.
- Cradle the telephone between your shoulder and chin.
- Prop your chin on one or both hands for extended periods.
- Reach high overhead to do work, like painting or hammering on walls or ceilings.
- Carry a heavy shoulder bag with a strap on the same shoulder for a long time.
- Wear high-heeled shoes.
- Yawn like the MGM lion. If you feel a yawn coming, stifle or restrain it by holding a fist under your chin.

Other experts have added their own do's and don'ts to the list of habits you should avoid or adopt if you want to combat TMJ:

Don't sleep with a pillow.   Instead, tuck yourself in with a thin towel rolled up under your neck (to about the thickness of your wrist). Place another towel under your back and a pillow under your knees. Sleeping in this position—on your back throughout the entire night—can be very relaxing to your jaws and "critical" to overcoming TMJ, says Owen J. Rogal, D.D.S., executive director of the American Academy of Head, Facial, and Neck Pain, and TMJ Orthopedics. But what if you generally sleep on your side? He suggests placing a beanbag on either side of your head to stop you from rolling over into that position.

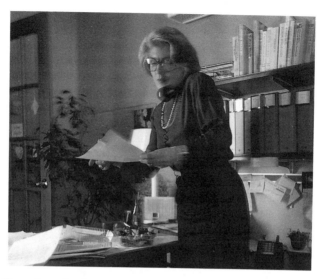

Cradling the telephone between your shoulder and chin is a nasty habit you should break if you want to relieve temporomandibular joint (TMJ) pain. Try using a headset for extended calls—it will allow you to free your hands without straining your jaw muscles.

Don't grind your teeth. There's little question that gnashing teeth, referred to by doctors as bruxism, can bring about or exacerbate TMJ troubles. Those who grit and grind usually do so because they're stressed. (Some say that clenching in reaction to stress or anger is a primal instinct.)

To combat TMJ, you should develop the habit of keeping your teeth slightly apart with the lips lightly touching.

Your teeth should touch only when you're chewing food or swallowing. If you practice keeping your teeth apart, it will reduce the urge to clench or grind. Set little reminders in key places around your home and office so that you won't forget. Or try repeating the phrase "lips together, teeth apart" as a reminder.

Unfortunately, clenching sometimes occurs during sleep, when it's hard to control. If you suspect that you're a night clencher, you might try wearing a mouth guard to bed. Sporting goods stores sell mouth guards that you put in hot water and then pop into your mouth and bite down on for a better fit. These inexpensive aids may be used temporarily to guard against night-time chomping—they will hold your jaws steady and may temporarily control your symptoms. If it works, tell your dentist. He can then make you a custom-fitted device.

Above all else, calm down. Experts agree that bruxism is most often related to stress, so the best thing you can do to stop clenching is to relax. Take it easy. Be gentle with yourself. Take warm baths and learn some good relaxation techniques such as progressive relaxation and meditation.

Instant Relief for Jaw-Breaking Pain

These three steps may help you stop your jaw pain on the spot.

First, take two buffered aspirin four times a day.

Next, do anything you can to increase blood flow to the area. You may want to apply moist heat or ice to the sides of your jaws. Heat works best for some, ice for others. You should experiment to see what works best for you.

With a warm or cold washcloth or ice pack in place over your jaws, you might try giving your jaws a brisk massage. The added rubbing action will help relax clenched jaw muscles and stimulate circulation in the area.

Third, wiggle your jaw joint periodically to work out tension. Exercise is another easy way to get blood flowing to the area. Bring your lower jaw forward and up in front of your upper jaw. Repeat ten times, twice a day.

Symptoms That Call for a Doctor's Care

The most common signs of a TMJ—among them headaches and popping noises when opening and closing your mouth—are usually nothing more than minor to moderate annoyances that will go away when the condition is corrected. Some symptoms, however, are considered serious and should be investigated by your doctor. If you can't open your mouth, can't brush your teeth, and are having sharp headaches, go see a doctor. Your TMJ may be getting worse.

Soothing a Bad Back

Olga Korbut's back sang of suppleness and grace as she arched toward the floor. Peggy Fleming's dazzled as she extended over the ice, back and leg one continuous line in a breathtaking spin. Mikhail Baryshnikov's conveys power as he executes a leap.

What a beautifully expressive part of the body the back can be. Yet it's capable of some not-so-beautiful expressions, too. Dull aches. Shooting pains. Prolonged agony.

An estimated eight out of every ten Americans will suffer from at least one episode of back pain in their lives. Indeed, back pain is the number one cause of disability for people under age 45 and the number three cause for people 45 and older.

And the incidence of back pain is on the rise. In fact, reports of back pain have increased 14 times faster than the population itself, says David Lehrman, M.D., founder and director of the Lehrman Back Care Center in Miami, and chief of orthopedic surgery at St. Francis Hospital. He thinks he may know why.

"Our grandparents spent their days exercising and being active—chopping wood, tilling the soil," he says. "These motions work the back, knees, hips, and arms to bring about balance in the body system. Today, as executives and office workers, we're doing more straining than strengthening of muscles. Sedentary lives lead to muscular imbalance.''

Muscle sprain or spasm is the most common cause of back pain. People who use their muscles frequently—day laborers, athletes—sometimes tend to suffer from back pain. But people who make a heavy demand on these muscles every once in a while—weekend athletes and employees whose jobs require occasional lifting—might be in for extra trouble.

Too much demand on a weak muscle can cause it to spasm, which is your body's way of saying, ''Cool out. If you push me beyond my limits, I'm going to tighten up so you can't do it again.'' Sometimes a group of muscles gets into the act, contracting in pain and immobilizing the injured area.

You experience that contraction as pain. As these contracted muscles tighten, the small blood vessels in them narrow, and that means less oxygen and nutrition from the blood get carried into the muscle cells and more wastes remain.

But just because your back is a target for a variety of aches doesn't mean that you have to baby it. In fact, the idea is to put your back to use. After all, your back was built for movement. Barring permanent disability, there's no reason not to jitterbug the night away or spend an afternoon digging in your garden.

''I think that one of the grossest misconceptions people have about the back is that it is vulnerable, weak, and easily injured,'' says John Sarno, M.D., a physiatrist and professor of clinical rehabilitation medicine at New York University's School of Medicine. ''That's not true. I always emphasize the strength and power of the back.''

To keep your back strong and powerful, experts advise the following: Exercise to keep your back muscles flexible. Learn to lift without injuring yourself. Sit, stand, and walk in ways that use the back as it was designed to be used.

Exercise to Keep Backache at Bay

Blame it all on progress. You didn't hear Cro-Magnon man complaining about his aching back. Before some now-forgotten inventor lashed some tree limbs together and designed the first chair, people either squatted or lay down when they needed to take a load off their feet. Both activities put far less pressure on the spine than sitting.

We sit for most of our 16 waking hours every day. Worse, a lot of us slouch in our chairs or sit hunched over work at a desk for long stretches of time.

All this sitting and slouching has resulted in stiff and weak muslces and a whole heap of back pain. And when you have slack muscles, even the smallest movements—bending down to pick up a paper clip, for example—can send your back into excruciating spasms.

This weakness in the musculature of the back has a name: myofascial syndrome. Myofascial refers to the muscles, ligaments, and connective tissues that support the vertebrae of the spine and wrap around the hips, buttocks, and stomach. "Myofascial syndrome is the source of more than 90 percent of all back pain," say Hubert Rosomoff, M.D., director of the University of Miami's Comprehensive Pain and Rehabilitation Center.

Work out the muscles that matter.   To have a pain-free back, you need to be sure that specific muscle groups are flexible and strong, says Dr. Rosomoff. In other words, you need to concentrate on exercises that stretch and strengthen the back extensor muscles (the ones along either side of the spine) and the muscles that encase your hip bones, buttocks, and upper legs.

You also need to pay particular attention to strengthening the abdominal muscles. How does fortifying the muscles in front of your body help your back? The answer is simple. The stomach muscles function much like guy wires of the back—they are the brace that keeps us upright. If they go slack, our back goes out of whack. When the stomach muscles are properly toned, however, they exert a pressure that helps support the front of the spine.

Stretch to combat stiffness.   To fortify your back, first focus on gentle stretching exercises that will help loosen up the muscles around your tailbone, hips, and hamstrings. (If you have undiagnosed back pain, check with your doctor or a physical therapist before doing these exercises.)

Try to work through the stiffness. The dull ache associated with exercise should start to subside by the third week. If you experience swelling, bruises, or sharp pain, however, stop immediately. These symptoms indicate pulled or torn muscles. Remember to use slow, steady motions and hold each pose at full range-of-motion for 6 seconds. Repeat the set of exercises at least twice a day. Gradually increase the number of sets, working both sides of your body.

Knee-to-chest: Lie on your back; bring both knees up to your chest. Grasp gently around your knees. Exhale slowly while you lift your head off the mat toward your knees. Hold 6 seconds; return feet to the mat.

Side-lying stretch: Lie on your side on the edge of a bed, facing the middle. Bend your bottom leg close to your chest. Keep your top leg straight at the hip and knee. Bring the top leg back behind the bottom leg. Allow it to dangle over the edge of the bed. Try to touch the floor. Do not arch your back. Bend the leg and return to starting position. Repeat, lying on your opposite side.

Hamstrings stretch: Lie on your back on the floor. Bend your right knee leaving your right foot flat on the floor. Now slowly and gently bring the left leg straight up, foot toward the ceiling. Hold this stretch 20 to 30 seconds. Repeat the exercise, bending the left knee and raising the right leg.

The best back strengtheners.   Part two of your back-building program is aimed at strengthening the muscles in your back, pelvis, and abdomen. Perform these simple exercises once a day:

Pelvic tilt: Lie flat on the floor with knees bent. Tighten your buttocks, pull in your stomach, and tilt your pelvis toward your face. Hold for 6 seconds. (Note: This exercise can also be performed while standing or sitting.)

Pray to Mecca: Kneel down, then sit back, resting your buttocks on your heels. Lower your torso and stretch your arms on the floor in front of you. Tuck your head down and pretend you are praying to Mecca. Now bring yourself back up on your hands and knees and slowly arch your back up like an angry cat. Hold, relax, and repeat.

Swim on dry land: Lie on your stomach and raise your left arm and your right leg. Hold for 1 second, then alternate with your left leg and right arm as if you were swimming.

Crunch sit-up: Lie on your back with your knees bent and both feet on the floor. Cross your arms and rest your hands on your shoulders. Raise your head and shoulders off the floor as high as you can while keeping your lower back on the floor. Hold for 1 second, then repeat.

Whatever you do, keep moving.   Studies have found that the people who are most immune to back pain are the most physically fit. A University of Copenhagen study of 105 backache sufferers found that long-term regular exercise offered the most improvement by far. And in another study, people who were the most fit were ten times less likely to develop back pain as those with the lowest levels of fitness.

Walking is a great way to keep your spine supple and strong. Cycling is good too, provided you raise the handlebars to a more upright position so you are not stooped over.

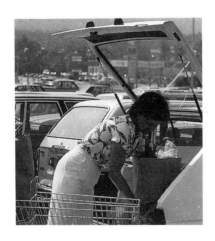

The back-saving way to lift groceries from your car trunk is to slide the groceries close to you, keep your spine straight, and bend your knees and waist—not your back.

Nine Ways to Relieve a Back Attack

Ninety percent of people who suffer an acute episode of back pain feel better within a week, says Stanley Herring, M.D., a Seattle physiatrist and University of Washington clinical assistant professor of rehabilitation medicine and orthopedics. What's more, physicians who specialize in back care say that even chronic back pain is treatable.

The following measures can get your spine feeling ship-shape. Remember, however, that once you've gotten rid of acute pain, you must identify what triggered your back attack. Once you identify the weaknesses, you can gradually begin to strengthen the affected areas or learn how to move in ways that don't add further injury. A back-care expert can help you tailor a program of exercise and posture correction for your body.

1. Curl up and lie on the floor.   The next time you feel that a lower backache is coming on but it's not quite debilitating yet, lie on your back and lift your legs up—carefully—onto the seat of a chair. Support your head and neck with a thin pillow. If you can assume this position within 5 to 10 minutes of the first backache twinge, your backache should be much milder than usual or disappear completely.

2. Stretch to smooth a spasm.   "Stretching will help the muscle calm down sooner than just waiting for it to calm down on its own," says Dr. Lehrman. One good stretch for lower back pain is to lie on a bed and gently bring your knees up to your chest. Once there, put a little pressure on your knees by cupping your hands over your knees and pulling them toward your chest. Then relax. Repeat.

3. Put your pain on ice.   The best way to cool down an acute flare-up is with ice. It will help reduce swelling and the strain on your back muscles. For best results, try ice massage. Put an ice pack on the site of the pain and massage the spot for 7 or 8 minutes. Do this for a day or two.

4. Try some heat relief.   After the first day or two of ice, switch to heat, says Milton Fried, M.D., founder and director of the Milton Fried Medical Clinic in Atlanta, Georgia. Take a soft towel and put it in a basin of very warm water. Wring it well and flatten it so that there are no creases in it. Lie chest-down with pillows under your hips and ankles and fold the towel across the painful part of your back. Put some plastic wrap over that, then put a heating pad, turned on medium, on top of the plastic. If possible, place some weight on top that will create pressure, like a heavy telephone book. "This creates moist heat and will help reduce muscle spasms," says Dr. Fried.

5. Use heat *and* cold.   For those of you who can't make up your mind which feels better, it's okay to use both methods. Apply 30 minutes of ice, then 30 minutes of heat, and keep repeating the cycle.

6. Try a self-massage.   Take two tennis balls and lie down on your back. Slide the tennis balls under the small of your back, one on each side of your spine. Take a deep breath and relax. Slowly work the tennis balls up your back. You can vary the pressure by simply shifting your weight around. Rub your whole back for 10 minutes or spend 10 minutes in just one problem area. Don't continue massaging if the pain increases. This technique is for sudden back pain from muscle sprains or strains caused by overexertion—not disk or nerve problems.

7. Take an aspirin a day.   It can keep back pain away, claim the experts. Back pain is often accompanied by inflammation around the site of the pain, and simple over-the-counter anti-inflammatory drugs such as aspirin and ibuprofen can help take it away. (Acetaminophen is not as effective because it's not an anti-inflammatory drug.)

8. Bark up the right tree.   If you're looking for a natural anti-inflammatory, try some white willow bark, which can be found in capsule form in health food stores, says Dr. Fried. "It is a natural salicylate, the active ingredient that gives aspirin its anti-inflammatory power," says Dr. Fried. "Taken after meals, it shouldn't hurt your stomach, and it works very well on mild to moderate back pain. Those who suffer from ulcers and heartburn, however, should not use it."

9. Get into the pool.   Just walking against the water's resistance can produce an effect on stiff back muscles that's similar to a doctor's manipulation. Just make sure the water is warm before you step in.

When Rest Is Best

For the ooh-I-can't-stand-up back pain, your best bet is to sleep off your agony. In fact, resting may be the only thing you'll want to do. The least bit of effort—even getting up to go to the bathroom—may bring you pain. So don't fight your pain—go to bed and follow these guidelines:

Find your painless position.   Take the pressure off your back. Lie on your back with several pillows under your legs and your knees somewhat bent. If you lie on your side, put a pillow or small roll under your waist and a pillow between your legs. The pillow stops your leg from sliding forward and rotating your hips, which puts added pressure on your back. If you like lying on your stomach, put pillows under your belly to support your lower back.

Don't lounge too long.   "How long you stay in bed depends on the severity of your pain," says Edward Abraham, M.D., assistant clinical professor of orthopedics at the University of California, Irvine, College of Medicine. "If you're still in pain after two days, for example, an extra day in bed won't hurt. It's best, however, to get out of bed as quickly as possible. Let pain be your guide."

In other words, an extra week of bed rest won't necessarily take away the pain. Researchers found that for every week of bed rest, it takes two weeks to rehabilitate. At the University of Texas Health Science Center in San Antonio, scientists studied 203 patients who came into a walk-in clinic complaining of acute back pain. Some were told to rest for two full days and others were told to rest for seven days. There was no difference in the length of time it took the pain to diminish in either group. And those who got out of bed after two days got back to work a lot sooner.

Roll out of bed.   When you do have to get out of bed, doctors advise that you slide to the edge of the bed and let your legs come off the bed first. Doing so will act like a springboard, lifting your upper body straight up off the bed.

Putting Out the Fire of Heartburn

Drop this book. Run to the fridge. Prepare two bologna sandwiches with gobs of mayonnaise, and tomatoes, and peppers. Have some beer. Pull out that cold pizza from Friday night. Yum yum. Help yourself to some ice cream with chocolate sauce. Don't forget the coffee, extra cream. Down it all as fast as you can—then hurry back for more.

All done?

Good. Now we're ready to talk heartburn.

What's heartburn? Just hold on a couple of minutes and you'll know.

What causes heartburn? It could be a number of things, but in most cases, it's *acid reflux.* That is, some of the digestive juices normally found in your stomach back up out of your stomach into your esophagus, the pipe between your stomach and your mouth. These juices include hydrochloric acid, the corrosive substance used in industry to clean metal.

Whereas the stomach has a protective lining so that it doesn't succumb to the acid, the esophagus has no such lining. That's why upwardly mobile stomach acid burns, sometimes so badly that you may think you're suffering a heart attack.

What causes stomach juices to rise? You guessed it—that sharklike attack on the refrigerator is the most common cause. But it's not the only one.

Help from the Experts

Unfortunately, some people suffer from heartburn even without overindulging. For all of you sufferers who need to understand a little bit more about how heartburn works—and how to squelch the fire—we turn to the experts.

Don't stuff your face.   Your stomach may suffer from feeding frenzies. When there's too much food in the belly, stomach acids can be forced up into the esophagus. Fill the belly more, and you'll force up more acid. There can be many reasons for heartburn, but for the occasional sufferer it's usually eating too much food too fast, says Samuel Klein, M.D., assistant professor of gastroenterology at the University of Texas Medical Branch, Galveston.

Give up greasy foods.   If you've just knocked off a triple cheeseburger with fries and a double milkshake, that probably explains your pain. Greasy, fried, and fatty foods tend to sit in the stomach for a long time and foster surplus acid production. Avoidance of fatty meats and dairy products will almost certainly discourage repeat attacks.

Go easy on the caffeine.   Caffeinated drinks such as coffee, tea, and cola may irritate an already-inflamed esophagus. Caffeine also relaxes the sphincter muscle, the valve that keeps acid in your stomach.

Chuck the chocolate.   It's the number one food to avoid when you're suffering from heartburn. The reason? The sweet confection deals heartburn sufferers a double whammy: It's nearly all fat, and it contains caffeine.

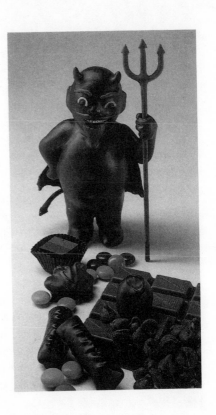

The combination of caffeine and fat makes chocolate the most sinister food for heartburn sufferers. If you must indulge in this sinful delight now and then, at least try white chocolate. While it's just as fatty, white chocolate has less caffeine than brown.

Swear off carbonated drinks. All those little bubbles can expand your stomach, having the same effect on the sphincter as overeating.

Go easy on hot sauce. Chili peppers and their spicy cousins may seem like the most likely heartburn culprits, but they're less of a problem than chocolate. Some heartburn sufferers can eat spicy foods without added pain, says Dr. Klein.

See if citrus fruits spell trouble. Acidic foods like oranges and lemons may seem like trouble, but the acid they contain is kid stuff compared to what your stomach produces. Let your tummy decide on these foods.

Don't rely on milk or mints. Mints are one of several

foods that tend to relax your lower esophageal sphincter, or LES, the little lid that can often protect you even when you do overindulge.

And what's wrong with milk? It's this: Fats, proteins, and calcium in milk can stimulate the stomach to secrete acid. "Some people recommend milk for heartburn—but there's a problem with it," says Dr. Klein. "It feels good going down, but it does stimulate acid secretion in the stomach."

Beer, wine, other alcoholic beverages, and tomatoes can also relax your sphincter, and should be avoided.

Stop nighttime noshing.   "Never eat within 2½ hours before bedtime," says Francis S. Kleckner, M.D., a gastroenterologist in Allentown, Pennsylvania. A bulging stomach and gravity working together are a sure way to force stomach acid upward into the esophagus.

Let your belt out a notch.   Or switch to wearing suspenders to escape the pain of heartburn. The stomach may be compared to a tube of toothpaste, says Dr. Kleckner. If you squeeze the tube in the middle, something's going to come out of the top. Too much pressure around your middle can instigate the common cause of heartburn—stomach acid backing up into your esophagus, searing the tender tissues. "Many people can get relief from heartburn simply by wearing suspenders instead of a belt," he says.

Lift the right way.   If you bend at the stomach, you'll be compressing it, forcing acid upward. "Bend at the knees," says Dr. Kleckner. "It's not only a way to control acid, it's also better for your back."

Steer clear of smoky rooms.   "It doesn't matter whether it's yours or someone else's tobacco smoke—avoid it," says Dr. Kleckner. Smoke can relax your sphincter and increase acid production.

Lie on an incline.   If you stay upright, the acid in your stomach is more likely to stay in your stomach. "Water doesn't travel uphill, and acid doesn't either," says Dr. Kleckner.

When you finally do lie down, elevate the head of your bed 4 to 6 inches. To do that, place blocks under the legs of the bed itself or slip a wedge under the mattress at the head of the bed. (Extra pillows, however, cannot be expected to do the trick.) Keeping the bed on a slant will discourage the heartburn from returning.

Suspect your medications.   A number of prescription drugs, including some antidepressants and sedatives, may aggravate heartburn. If you're suffering heartburn and are on any prescription drug, "review it with your physician," says Dr. Kleckner.

How Do You Spell Relief?
H-E-R-B-S

Walk into your favorite health food store and chances are you'll find for sale a number of herbs that are reputed to fight heartburn. Daniel B. Mowrey, Ph.D., author of The Scientific Validation of Herbal Medicine, has looked at the evidence thoroughly and has come to the conclusion that, yes, some herbal remedies do relieve and prevent heartburn.

- **Gingerroot.** This, says Dr. Mowrey, is the most helpful. "I've seen it work often enough that I'm convinced," he says. "We're not sure how it works, but it seems to absorb the acid and have the secondary effect of calming the nerves," he says. Take it in capsule form just after you eat. Start with two capsules and increase the dosage as needed. You know you've taken enough, says Dr. Mowrey, when you start to taste ginger in your throat.
- **Bitters.** A class of herbs called bitters, used for many years in parts of Europe, is also helpful,

Use antacids sparingly.   Over-the-counter digestive aids are generally effective and safe. One would hope so: Americans pay billions a year for these medications. The antacids that get the highest marks from experts are many of the most common names— all those whose labels say they're made from a mixture of magnesium hydroxide and aluminum hydroxide. (One constipates and the other tends to produce diarrhea; combined, they counter each other's side effects.)

One caution: Although the mix may be relatively free of side effects, it's not a good idea to stay on these antacids for more than

---

Dr. Mowrey says. Examples of common bitters are gentian root, wormwood, and goldenseal. "I can vouch that they work," says Dr. Mowrey. Bitters can be taken in capsule form or as a liquid extract just before you eat.

- **Aromatics.** The aromatic herbs, such as catnip and fennel, are also reputed to be good for heartburn, "but the research on these is sporadic," says Dr. Mowrey.

- **Apple-cider vinegar.** Outside the herb family, an oft-touted remedy for heartburn is a teaspoon of apple-cider vinegar in half of a glass of water sipped during a meal. "I've used it many times— it definitely works," says Betty Shaver, a lecturer on home remedies at the New Age Health Spa in Neversink, New York. It may sound bizarre to ingest an acid when you have an acid problem, admits Shaver, but "there are good acids and bad acids," she says.

a month or possibly two, says Dr. Kleckner. They are so effective that they could be masking a serious problem that warrants a physician's care, he says.

Take it easy.   "Stress," says Dr. Klein, "may cause an increase in acid production in the stomach. Some good relaxation techniques might be of help in reducing your level of tension, allowing you to rebalance your unbalanced body chemistry."

Reduce stomach flab.   Think again of the toothpaste analogy, says Dr. Kleckner. A roll of fat around the gut squeezes the stomach much as a hand would squeeze a tube of toothpaste. But what you get is stomach acid.

Is It Heartburn or an Ulcer?

If you're experiencing heartburn regularly—two or three times a week for more than a month—for no apparent reason, it's time to call your doctor. Your pain may be a sign of an ulcer.

In addition, know that heartburn caused by simple acid reflux is normally worse after meals. If your heartburn worsens before meals, it may be a sign of an ulcer.

Heartburn accompanied by any of the following symptoms should be checked out by a physician *fast*. It could mean you're having a heart attack.

- Difficulty or pain when swallowing
- Vomiting with blood
- Bloody or black stool
- Shortness of breath
- Dizziness or light-headedness
- Pain radiating into your neck and shoulder

13 Ways to Quell Menstrual Cramps

Some women sail through their menstrual cycle without skipping a beat. Others have to skip out on their regular routine to deal with the pain and misery of menstrual cramps.

What causes cramps? One theory is that some women produce excess amounts of prostaglandins (hormonelike substances made from essential fatty acids, mentioned in earlier chapters) at the onset of their periods. The prostaglandins help the uterine muscles contract and expel tissue and fluids during menstruation. High levels of prostaglandins cause uterine muscle contractions, or cramps.

But you need not be sidelined by menstrual cramping each month. The following remedies could relieve the discomfort.

1. Limit junk food. "Too many women tend to skip meals and consume excessive amounts of sweets and salty foods just at a time when they should be so careful in their dietary choices," says Penny Wise Budoff, M.D., who runs a women's medical center in Bethpage, New York, and who is author of *No More Menstrual Cramps and Other Good News*.

While a healthier diet won't cure cramps, it can do wonders for improving your overall sense of well-being. Cut out salty and sweet junk foods, which can make you feel bloated and sluggish. Instead, eat more vegetables, fruits, chicken, and fish, and try to space them out in small meals throughout the day rather than having three large meals.

2. Take multivitamins multiple times.   Many of her patients report fewer problems with cramps when they're getting a healthy daily dose of vitamins and minerals, says Dr. Budoff. Take a multiple vitamin and mineral supplement, preferably one that comes in small doses that you can take a couple of times a day after meals, she advises.

3. Put minerals on your menu.   The minerals calcium, potassium, and magnesium can also play a part in relief, says Susan Lark, M.D., director of the PMS Self-Help Center in Los Altos, California. She says she has found that women taking calcium suffer less pain from cramps than those who do not. Magnesium is important, she notes, because it helps your body absorb calcium more efficiently. She suggests increasing calcium and magnesium intake before and during your period.

4. Go caffeine-free.   The caffeine in coffee, tea, cola, and chocolate can contribute to menstrual discomfort by making you nervous, says Dr. Budoff. Kick the caffeine habit. The oils in coffee also may irritate your intestines.

5. Cut back on booze.   If you tend to retain water during your period, alcohol will only add to your problem. If you must drink, limit yourself to a glass or two of light wine.

6. Reduce bloating naturally.   Many women think diuretics are great for reducing menstrual bloating, but Dr. Lark advises against them. Diuretics have the ability to take important minerals from the body along with the water. Instead, she advises, reduce your intake of water-retentive substances like salt and alcohol.

7. Cozy up to a heating pad.   Warmth will increase your blood flow and relax your muscles—especially important in your cramped and congested pelvic area, says Dr. Budoff. Place a heating pad or hot water bottle on your abdomen for a few minutes at a time. And be sure to drink lots of hot herbal tea or hot lemonade.

8. Take to your tub.   A nice warm bath will increase your blood flow and relax your muscles to relieve the cramps. For a tingling effervescent effect, choose bath salts that contain sodium bicarbonate, or baking soda.

9. Take a brisk walk.   When you are in pain—or anticipate pain—you tend to contract your muscles involuntarily and hold your breath, says Dr. Lark. But shallow breathing and tight muscles can decrease the amount of blood flow and oxygen to the tissues and aggravate menstrual pain.

Regular workouts like walking, tennis, and swimming can improve breathing and blood flow and help to prevent the fluid retention and swelling in body tissues that can make you feel achy.

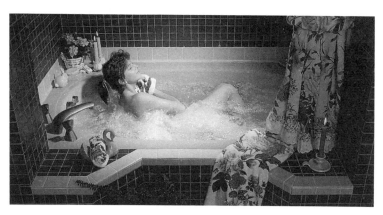

Create your own relaxing health spa for easing monthly cramps. Simply add 1 cup of sea salt and 1 cup of baking soda to a warm bath. The warmth increases blood flow and relaxes your muscles to reduce the cramps, while the added minerals soften your skin. Toss in a sprig of lavender for a heavenly scent.

10. Curl up in a ball.   The yoga position known as the child's pose can be a great way to stretch out cramp spasms. All you do is sit back on your heels with your arms limp at your sides. Bring your forehead to the floor, and place your arms along the floor against your body. Close your eyes. Hold the position for as long as it is comfortable.

11. Have a backrub.   According to women's athletic trainer Bill Prentice, Ph.D., of the University of North Carolina, a massage can rub away minor cramps. Ask a friend to use fingers or thumb and firmly rub in circles at the midsection of your back, just right of the third bony vertebra up from the base of your spine. The pain may disappear in less than five minutes.

12. Make love.   Having sex with orgasm is great for relieving cramps, says Dr. Lark. The vigorous muscle action moves blood and other fluids away from congested organs, relieving pain.

13. Take an OTC.   Aspirin and acetaminophen are fine for relieving cramps. Even more effective, however, are over-the-counter medications like Advil, Medipren, Haltran, and Nuprin, says Dr. Budoff. These contain ibuprofen, which has the ability to inhibit the actions of prostaglandins. Take one of these medications—along with some milk or food to avoid stomach irritation—when your cramps start and continue taking them until the cramps go away.

Diet and Exercise: The Modern Prescription for Arthritis

Unfortunately, joints don't come with a lifetime guarantee. Like other major organs, the joints and soft tissues around them are vulnerable to an array of mishaps and maladies. Any part of a joint can become overstressed or affected by disease. The result? "Fire in the joints." That is what the word "arthritis" means—and what arthritis feels like—to millions of Americans.

The fiery pain is caused by inflammation, the common symptom of the two main kinds of arthritis. Osteoarthritis is a wear-and-tear disease that affects people as they age: Bone cartilage wears down, triggering inflammation of the surrounding joint. People who suffer from this kind of arthritis frequently have stiffness, tenderness, and a deep, aching pain in one or more joints, especially those that bear weight, such as the hips, knees, and feet. Another form of osteoarthritis targets the hands, causing knobby enlargements of the finger joints and pain at the base of the thumb.

Rheumatoid arthritis, on the other hand, can strike young and old. It's a whole-body disease in which the immune system attacks the body's own tissues. Joint inflammation is just one symptom.

These are just two forms of arthritis. There are actually more than 100 other types of arthritis-related diseases, and the list of potential causes is mind-boggling. Infections, injuries, overuse, heredity, stress, and even food allergies have all been implicated in some kinds of arthritis.

Regardless of the cause, though, the end result of arthritis is often the same: stiff, painful, swollen, and inflamed joints.

Although there is no cure for arthritis, a variety of medications are prescribed to alleviate the inflammation and pain, such as aspirin and ibuprofen. While these drugs are a boon to arthritis sufferers, they can have side effects. So it makes sense to get by with as little medication as possible.

You *can* fight back against painful, swollen joints. The correct balance of diet, exercise, and relaxation can dramatically relieve arthritis pain and inflammation.

Anatomy of the Anti-Arthritis Diet

One way to cut down on the need for medication may be to follow a diet that reduces inflammation. There is now scientific evidence that what you eat may make a difference in quenching the fires of both major types of arthritis. (Just be sure to discuss any changes in diet or medication with your physician before taking action.)

Fighting fire with fish oil.   Fish oils have a unique group of ''fatty acids''(a technical term for a biological component of fat) that scientists have dubbed omega-3's. Research shows that omega-3's may help reduce the inflammation of rheumatoid arthritis.

How does this type of fatty acid quench the flames? For starters, inflammation of arthritis is caused by prostaglandins, hormonelike substances that are produced from yet another type of fatty acids—the omega-6's—which are found in certain foods we eat. Most vegetable oils are rich in omega-6-type fatty acids such as linoleic acid and arachidonic acid. It's these fatty acids that help to create the inflammatory prostaglandin.

There is now evidence that these pain-producing prostaglandins have less chance of giving you trouble if you eat adequate amounts of foods rich in the omega-3's. Apparently, in the body, the good-guy omega-3 fatty acids compete with the bad-guy omega-6 fatty acids to create a different type of prostaglandin that does not trigger inflammation.

This fatty acid duel is illustrated in the results of one notable study. Researchers examined the effects of fish oil on the symptoms of 33 patients with mild to severe rheumatoid arthritis. Before the study began, all the subjects endured morning stiffness for longer than 30 minutes and had multiple swollen and tender joints. For 14 weeks, half the group took 15 fish-oil supplement capsules a day, while the other half took placebos (harmless look-alikes); then the groups switched for another 14 weeks.

Results: When the people took fish oil, they experienced a third less joint tenderness than when they took a placebo.

Researchers say that more studies need to be conducted before any new recommendations on adding fish or fish-oil supplements to the diet can be made with a higher degree of confidence.

In the meantime, "It's irrefutable that eating more fish is a healthy step for any person, arthritis or not," says Joel M. Kremer, M.D., associate professor of medicine, Albany Medical College. "In our studies, the doses of fish oil given were roughly equal to a salmon dinner or a can of sardines," Dr. Kremer explains. "If you've got arthritis now, you can use traditional therapies for relief and also continue to eat more fish. It certainly won't hurt, and may help your inflammation."

Deep-sea fish is your best catch.   To get more omega-3 oil, make fish a regular part of your diet. In particular, select the oil-rich, deep-water fish, such as salmon, tuna, halibut, and sardines (packed in water, not in vegetable oil). There are other sources of omega-3's as well, most notably walnuts, soybeans, and tofu. But none delivers as much of this inflammation-fighting oil as deep-water fish do.

Find a better way to dress your salad.   At the same time you are increasing your consumption of the omega-3 foods, you should decrease foods that contain the harmful omega-6's—namely, vegetable oils such as safflower, corn, sunflower, and so on. Nix salad dressings, fried foods, margarine, and other related foods that may consist of vegetable oils. You don't have to strike oil completely from your menu, however. An alternative is to switch to canola oil, made from rapeseed, and olive oil: These two oils are low in the bad-guy omega-6's.

Lean toward lean.   Saturated fat—the kind of fat found in red meat and dairy products—should be on your list of bad fats you should banish from your menu—or at least limit if you suffer from arthritis.

In a study conducted by Charles P. Lucas, M.D., clincal professor of medicine at Wayne State University School of Medicine in Detroit and director of the Division of Preventive and Nutritional Medicine at William Beaumont Hospital in Birmingham, Michigan, people with rheumatoid arthritis dramatically improved when they stopped eating high-fat dairy products and meat.

Dr. Lucas believes the reduction in dietary fats reduces the production of prostaglandins, the hormonelike substances that trigger inflammation.

So do your joints a favor. Trade your red-meat meals for more fish and poultry. Find new recipes for meatless entrées. Ease off the whole milk and cheese and stock up on skim milk, yogurt, part-skim mozzarella, and low-fat cottage cheese. If you want to butter your bread—why not try a fruit butter instead. You'll get lip-smacking flavor without the saturated fat. Remember to cook lighter, too. Steaming, baking, and broiling without fat are better than frying.

Have some oranges and ease achy joints.   Oranges and other citrus fruits as well as tomatoes, strawberries, green peppers, and mustard greens are chock-full of vitamin C. And, according to some studies, people with rheumatoid arthritis are deficient in vitamin C, says Robert H. Davis, Ph.D., professor of physiology at the Pennsylvania College of Podiatric Medicine. Dr. Davis's medical models have shown that a lack of vitamin C can aggravate

Fewer Pounds, Less Pain

Eating a low-fat diet can help relieve your arthritis in two ways: You'll reduce inflammation and you'll lose weight. When you shed extra pounds, you reduce stress on your aching joints, especially if you have arthritis in weight-bearing joints such as your knees, back, or hips.

In fact, studies show that being overweight can actually cause arthritis of the knee. That conclusion was drawn from information from the ongoing Framingham Heart Study in Massachusetts. Boston University researchers studied two groups of older Framingham citizens, with and without arthritis of the knee. When the researchers looked at data from when the people were in their midthirties, they found that those—particularly women— with arthritis had been significantly heavier than those without the problem.

rheumatoid arthritis and that strong doses of vitamin C can bring about regression of the disease.

The Recommended Dietary Allowance of vitmain C is about 60 milligrams. But you may consider supplements. ''Vitamin C is definitely a good home remedy for someone with rheumatoid arthritis,'' he says. ''The toxicity of vitamin C is virtually zero, and if a person took about 500 milligrams spread throughout the day, which is not excessive, that would get enough of the vitamin through to do some good.'' Before trying vitamin C therapy, get an okay from your doctor.

Have a cup of skim milk a day.   That's one way to help meet your calcium quota. (The Recommended Dietary Allowance for calcium is 800 milligrams for adults.) While everyone needs to get enough calcium in his diet, people with rheumatoid arthritis should be doubly careful because they are more likely to lose calcium from their bones, especially if they take corticosteroid medications. When the bones lose calcium, they become porous and fragile, a conditon known as osteoporosis. And this brittle-bone disease can add to the aches and pains of many people with arthritis.

Besides milk, other good calcium-rich sources are cheese, dark leafy greens, canned sardines, tofu, soybeans, broccoli, and legumes.

Moving Away from Pain

Nowhere is the adage "use it or lose it" more apropos than with arthritis. "The longer you sit around in pain doing nothing, the worse it gets," says Michele Boutaugh, B.S.N., Arthritis Foundation vice president for patient services. "You get stiffer and stiffer, and eventually you can lose the use of the affected joint." As the joints become stiff, the muscles don't work as hard, and they weaken through disuse. Weak muscles, in turn, increase the risk of injury to the joint and can aggravate arthritis.

A careful exercise program helps to build up bones, strengthen muscles, and keep joints "well oiled" and gliding smoothly—an important factor in combating osteoarthritis. In this form of arthritis, the cartilage becomes frayed so bones grate against joints, especially in the weight-bearing joints like hips and knees. Using your joints can actually smooth off or polish these rough edges and keep the joints working more smoothly.

What else does exercise do? For one thing, it acts as a natural pain reliever. In several studies, arthritic patients who walked, rode stationary bikes, danced, or did swimming pool exercises actually reduced their pain and swelling. With regular exercise, some people felt so much better that they needed less medication.

Perhaps the most exciting news about exercise's benefits for arthritis is the evidence that shows that it may actually slow the progress of rheumatoid arthritis. In one 8-year study, researchers found that among people who had this disease, those who kept up with daily exercise over the years spent only half as much time in the hospital as the inactive group.

The Range-of-Motion Exercises

Some people believe that the word "exercise" includes normal daily activities, such as housework, climbing stairs, bending and lifting, or walking. These activities may maintain and improve endurance and muscle tone, and are fine. But there are some special exercises quite unlike any others, exercises that work specifically on joints. These are the range-of-motion exercises that are the backbone of your exercise program. Range-of-motion exercises help keep joints loose, improve muscle strength, and help restore movement that's been lost. Here are some common ones:

For aching hips.   Lie on your back with legs straight and about 6 inches apart. Point your toes up. Slide one leg out to the side and then back. Try to keep your toes pointing up, then repeat the exercise with your other leg.

For shoulder stiffness.   A good range-of-motion exercise for arthritis in the shoulders is to stay on your back and raise one arm over your head, keeping your elbow straight. Keep your arm close to your ear. Return your arm slowly to your side, and repeat the movement with your other arm.

(Your physician or therapist will be able to give you more exercises specifically suited to the parts of your body affected by arthritis.)

Move inch by inch.   When doing any of these range-of-motion exercises, move the joint until you feel some pain, hold it there a moment, then move it a wee bit farther. If there's slight pain in the joint, be gentle as you move it through whatever motion is possible. Sometimes you may need help, but try to perform as many as possible yourself. If you have a helper, he shouldn't use force when helping you with the movements. If possible, do 5 to 10 repetitions per exercise.

Maintain a proper pace.   Begin at a comfortable level and gradually increase the number of repetitions to avoid unnecessary pain. Use slow and steady rhythms, relax your muscles for about 10 to 15 seconds between repetitions, and breathe deeply and rhythmically as you exercise. Do not hold your breath.

Strengthening Joints Is a Must

No exercise program to soothe arthritic pain would be complete without strengthening exercises. The reason? Weak muscles add to joint problems. Flabby muscles perform like worn-out shock absorbers. They can't cushion the impact of movements, so the bones and cartilage absorb more shock than usual. Bones develop tiny fractures, and cartilage changes may lead to osteoarthritis.

Fortunately, you don't need to bulk up or become a power lifter to build stronger muscles. In fact, most physical therapists advise against working out with weights, as this may overstress weakened joints. A better idea: isometric exercises. These exercises (in which you press one muscle or part of the body against another or against an immovable object using a strong but motionless flexing action) have the advantage of causing little joint stress. Here are two isometrics to try:

Wall push-ups.   Place your hands on a wall and push. You can feel your arm muscles working, but there's no joint movement.

Knee press.   Sit in a chair and place your right hand on your right knee. Press your knee against your hand while allowing no movement of the arm and leg.

You need not do many isometric exercises to receive the benefits. Each routine held for a count of 6 seconds, three to four times a day, is enough.

Eight Ways to Limber Up Safely

If you're one of the people who suffer from arthritis and you're eager to begin an exercise program, don't run out and start doing something strenuous like jumping jacks. "Before you start exercising, check with your physician," says Frederic C. McDuffie, M.D., vice president of medical affairs for the Arthritis Foundation. "Too much exercise can be as harmful as too little. Your doctor can help you design a program specifically for your needs."

Once you have your doctor's blessing, your exercise program will be successful if you keep the following in mind:

1. Establish a routine time and place.   Some people find that exercising first thing in the day reduces their morning stiffness. Once you find a suitable time to exercise, make a commitment to work out each day.

2. Exercise when you are in the least pain.   If you're taking a prescription pain medication, plan to do your workout when the drug is having the most effect. Even if there's slight pain, you need to do the range-of-motion exercises to keep your joints loose. If the joint is hot, inflamed, swollen, red, or tender to the touch, move it gently through its range of motion. If in doubt, contact your doctor or therapist to find out how to adapt your exercises.

3. Cushion your feet from shock.   Wear shock-absorbent shoes. And work out on a surface with a little give. Ground or wood flooring puts less stress on joints than a concrete surface.

4. Apply warmth before your workout.   You can apply mild heat (hot isn't necessary) to help relax joints and muscles. It can be a warm bath or whirlpool, a shower or hand-held massage unit so you can aim the water at painful joints, an electric heating pad, a hot-water bottle, or hot packs. You can even stand next to a heater or radiator. In any case, about 20 minutes should be enough in most cases to prime your joints for exercise.

If you find that cold offers better relief than heat, try applying a plastic bag of ice to your affected joint for about 10 to 15 minutes.

5. Avoid drafts.   Chilly air can cause muscles and joints to stiffen. Wear warm clothing and don't exercise in a drafty or cold room.

6. Begin and end with a stretch.   You must get your body—specifically your aching joints—slowly prepared for exercise, so make stretching the first step before each workout. Here's one example of a safe, slow stretch: While lying in bed, stretch one arm up and then the other. Push your arms forward while opening your hands wide, then pull your arms back and close your hands. For your legs, pull your knees up toward your midsection, do a few slow bicycle turns, then stretch your legs out straight.

To avoid injury and reduce stiffness or soreness the next day, it's a good idea to stretch as part of your cooling-down process each time you finish exercising.

7. Listen to your body.   When you've finished for the day, you may feel a bit sore. If there's so much pain that you need medication after each workout, modify your program. Pain that persists is a sign that you're overdoing things or that there's something mechanically wrong in the joint.

If exercise-induced pain lasts longer than two hours or if the next day your symptoms are worse in the joints you exercised, then you've done too much. Next time cut back or exercise less strenuously. If necessary, find a different exercise that will give you the same results.

8. Know when to stop.   Do not continue exercising if you have tightness or pain in your chest, shortness of breath, dizziness, muscle pain or cramping, or if you're suddenly sick to your stomach. Another signal to stop is extremely sharp pain or more pain than normal—your body is giving you a warning.

First Aid for Flare-Ups

Your joints are sizzling and you feel as stiff as the Tin Man in the Wizard of Oz. But you've got things to do, people to see, places to go. Don't let your arthritis stop you. Here is how you can bring about pain relief without getting a prescription filled or making a trip to the doctor.

Quench the fire with cold water.   Cold temporarily numbs the pain and reduces the swelling from rheumatoid arthritis. Soak hot, swollen, painful joints of your hands or feet in a bucket or sink of cold water (around 65°F) for 15 to 20 minutes. Or place an ice pack on tender joints periodically throughout the day.

Some like it hot.   If your joint or muscle is *not* actively inflamed, hot, swollen, and red, apply heat. A heating pad or hot water bottle (wrapped in a towel) or a stream of shower water can

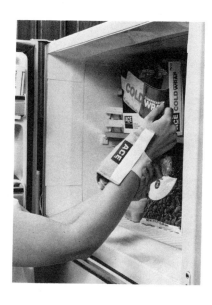

Studies show that placing an ice bag on arthritic joints for 20 minutes three times a day can ease pain, reduce stiffness, and help you reduce pain medication. You don't need a fancy ice pack. Just keep a bag of frozen peas handy, slam it against the counter and—voilà—you have a malleable pack ready for soothing fiery joints.

help limber up stiff joints and relieve pain by relaxing tense muscles, thus relieving pressure on the joints.

Try hot and cold.   You may find the contrast of alternating between warm and cold treatments most effective in relieving arthritis pain. To take a contrast bath, fill one container with warm water and another with cool water. Put your hands or feet in the warm water for 3 minutes, then switch to the cool water for 1 minute. Repeat this procedure two or three times, ending with warm water.

Use a dehumidifier.   Lowering household humidity may stop arthritis pain caused by weather changes. When rain is on the way, increases in air pressure and humidity can affect blood flow to arthritic joints, says Joseph Hollander, M.D., professor emeritus of medicine at the University of Pennsylvania. The areas can become stiff, swollen, and painful, but usually improve once the storm starts.

Try a whole-hand massage.   To help relieve aching, arthritic hands, start by slowly opening and closing them, then rub the palms together in a circular motion. Keep the fingers of one hand together, then squeeze and press them with the other hand. Spread the fingers, then gently squeeze and pull each one. Then, using a lubricating lotion, rub several times from the wrist to the fingertips and back again. Then stroke the forearm, rubbing toward the elbow and back, squeezing the muscles like a sponge. Repeat with the other hand. Pain relief comes from both the warmth and the increased blood circulation you generate with massage.

Rent a TENS.   Transcutaneous Electrical Nerve Stimulation (TENS, for short) uses a portable, battery-powered gadget with electrodes that you attach to your skin at the site of a painful joint. You adjust the electrical pulses for just the right voltage and frequency to stop your pain. TENS may work by blocking pain messages to the brain or by stimulating production of morphine-like endorphins, or both. With a doctor's prescription, you can rent a TENS unit for a one-month trial.

You may need to consider a new drug.   If these natural relief measures fail to soothe your arthritic pain, and if other over-the-counter anti-inflammatory drugs like aspirin or ibuprofen haven't doused the fire, ask your doctor about the newer inflammation-reducing drugs. Misoprostol is one that seems to prevent and even heal the side effects associated with prolonged use of aspirin.

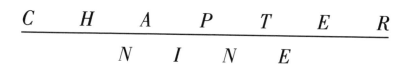
On-the-Spot Aid for Sprains and Strains

You're two pages into typing a letter to your sister, and the aching tingle in your wrists makes you want to give up your correspondence.

It's the second day of your hiking trip. As you're trekking down a steep trail, you let out a sharp cry of pain. You clutch your cramped calf.

You've exercised almost every Saturday. You've played rousing games of racquetball, tennis, and basketball; but still you find you have sore hamstrings, a strained shoulder, and, sometimes, shinsplints.

Whether you let your feet jump around the tennis court or you let your fingers walk over the keyboard, the same motion over and over has given you a pain.

In other words, you are a victim of repeated stressful movements—of doing too much, too often. What parts of our bodies take the biggest licking from overuse? The muscles and tendons in our wrists, shoulders, back, knees, thighs, and ankles. All these areas can be strained, sprained, pulled, wrenched, or cramped.

The affected area feels tender and will soon begin to swell. Probably by morning you will feel painfully stiff.

That doesn't have to be the end of your particular activity, however. Nor do you have to suffer through the achiness for hours or days. Below you will find a number of first-aid tips to ease those stop-in-your-tracks jolts of pain, whether you've incurred a cramp, a strain, or general soreness.

Follow Guidelines for Self-Treatment

If you are confused about when you should treat soreness on your own, read on.

Much everyday soreness results from *strains,* which means you have overstretched—or pulled—a muscle. *Sprains* are also quite common, but can be a bit more serious. This injury means you have either wrenched or twisted a ligament around a joint and that you may also have damaged some muscles, tendons, or nerves. If you have a mild to moderate sprain, you're likely to have limited function of the injured area, tenderness, possible muscle spasm, and painful range of motion. Swelling and discoloration may develop.

The general rule for treating sprains and strains is that if you hurt but can still walk and talk, try one of the standard self-treatments and then see how your injury responds in 48 hours. If the functioning of your injured area is still marginal after 24 to 72 hours, see your doctor. If you have a *severe* sprain—meaning you have loss of use in the affected body part, and there is much pain, tenderness, swelling, and discoloration—contact a doctor immediately.

As far as specific sprains, doctors say watch out for wrists. "Wrist sprains can be the most dangerous," says Thomas F. Griffin, Jr., M.D., medical director of the Douglas Clinic in Douglas, Arizona. "If your wrist pain lasts more than 48 hours, see a doctor, because the small wrist bones can disintegrate and cause a permanent dysfunction of the hand." For knees and ankles, the pain should subside in three days. If not, see your doctor. Also if you feel pain when bearing weight after 24 hours or you hear a popping or ripping in the joint or become unstable in the knee or ankle, see a doctor immediately.

RICE Is the First Rule

You probably know from experience that you don't have to be running a race to injure your muscles. Working in the yard, walking around the zoo all day, or simply sitting in an unfamiliar or awkward position, or in the same position for a long time, can cause muscle problems.

Whatever causes your injury, your muscles are going to let you know it in some way. More than likely there will be some swelling around your joints, which cuts off circulation and gives you a whopping pain. Stiffness may set in. Therefore, the primary first-aid treatment measure for sprains and strains is to reduce the swelling. Just remember the four-letter word RICE. The letters stand for Rest, applying an Ice pack, wrapping the injury with a Compress (such as an ace bandage), and Elevating the injured limb. All these methods will help reduce swelling so healing can take place. Here's a rundown of how RICE works to ease your pain.

Rest it.   It takes 48 hours for muscles to heal from exercise. Soreness means damage, and you should stop exercising when you feel sore. If you overdo any activity where you use your arms overhead—tennis or wall painting, for instance—you can cause painful tears and inflammation in your shoulder muscles.

How much rest you should give your muscles depends on the severity of the injury and the situation, says Allan Levy, M.D., director of the Department of Sports Medicine at Pascack Valley Hospital in New Jersey. A cramp may require only minutes of rest, a severe strain or sprain may need days or weeks. But sometimes you might not have the luxury of resting the muscle as long as needed. "If you're out hiking, for example, and strain a muscle, at least rest for a couple of hours before trying to continue," Dr. Levy advises. While you are resting, concentrate on applying other parts of the RICE rule.

Put yourself on ice.   Use an ice pack and apply it for 20 minutes at a time throughout the day.

Caution: Keep the ice off the affected area for at least as long as you keep it on. "The ice constricts your blood vessels, and it's not good to constrict your blood vessels too long," says Carol Folkerts, orthopedic coordinator of physical therapy at the University of Maryland Hospital in Baltimore. "You could kill the viable tissue in that area." People with heart disease, diabetes, and vascular diseases are especially vulnerable, and they should use ice with caution and only with the consent of their doctor.

Don't continue to apply ice directly to your skin after it begins to turn pink. For longer-lasting ice treatment, it's usually best to keep a layer of cloth between the ice and you.

Put your injury under wraps.   Don't make a mummy out of that sore calf or ankle, but wrap it in an Ace bandage to keep the swelling down. Just be careful not to wrap too tightly, or you could cause swelling below the injured area.

Fire up.   After applying ice to your injury, you may switch to heat for acute soreness or strain. Heat will dilate the blood vessels and promote healing.

Warm baths, whirlpools, and heating pads are all effective temporary pain relievers for soreness, strains, and cramps; but use discretion with heat treatments. A good rule is never apply heat in the first 48 hours after an injury or if there is swelling. With that in mind, if you have some stiffness two or three days after the injury, you can then soak it or warm it briefly to loosen it up. Simply wrap a hot, wet towel around the strain, cover with plastic wrap, and finish with a dry towel to hold in the heat. Apply hot packs four or five times a day for 20 minutes at a time. Caution: Tissue damage can occur if you rub any type of ointment on your skin before applying a hot pack. Don't use heat at all without a doctor's O.K. if your skin is heat sensitive due to poor circulation, diabetes, or steroid medications.

Raise your injury.   Raise your injured foot, lower leg, ankle, or wrist higher than your heart. This will prevent blood from pooling which causes swelling.

Pop a pain reliever.   In addition to RICE, you may want to try aspirin or ibuprofen. These medications will reduce pain and inflammation, whereas acetaminophen reduces pain but doesn't do anything for inflammation. Ibuprofen (Advil, Medipren, or Nuprin, for example) is the over-the-counter painkiller of choice because it reduces inflammation and provides pain relief without causing the stomach problems associated with aspirin.

Get a Move On

When you have mild or moderate muscle cramping or strains, you can counteract stiffness with gentle movements. Muscles injured during exercise shorten during the healing process, and unless the muscles are then lengthened, they will remain tight and more likely to be injured or torn. Here are a few guidelines for working your overworked muscles and tendons.

Str-e-t-c-h to unkink cramps.   For cramps and spasms, gradually stretch the muscle out and you'll get the muscle to relax. If the cramp is in your foot, pull your toes toward your face, for example. Stretching exercises can take care of your soreness as it exists now and prevent soreness in the future. (Instructions on stretching exercises follow, under the heading "Stretches to Keep Pain at Bay.")

Rotate your wrists.   If you have tingling in your wrist, it may be a symptom of carpal tunnel syndrome, a disease in which the nerve passing through the wrist is pinched by surrounding tissues, often caused by repeated movement of the wrists. To stop the numbing feeling, do several wrist circles. Then, try gentle squeezing motions of the fingers. Finally, press your fingers into your palm, then stretch them way back and hold. Repeat.

Tomorrow, repeat a slow version of your workout.   If you feel sore from an exercise workout, the rule is this: Take one day of rest, then do a shorter, lighter workout than usual. Repeat the one-day-off/one-day-easy sequence until all pain is gone. Moderate exercise can alleviate pain from overused muscles faster than inactivity. But listen to your body. If the pain gets worse when you continue to exercise, stop and see your doctor, says Robert D. Willix, Jr., sportsmedicine specialist and director of the Willix Health Institute.

Branch out.   This is perhaps an even better idea than the hard/easy routine. If you're suffering sore lower leg muscles or knee pain, for instance, try mixing in some swimming or bicycling (which works the upper legs) so you can continue exercising while healing. Swimming, biking, or rowing will not place great strain on the knees.

Stretches to Keep Pain at Bay

Give muscles the attention they need, and they tend to do their jobs quietly. Ignore them, and they'll grab your attention—or your leg, your arm, your shoulder, any part of you.

When that happens, you may be able to quiet them again with some simple stretching. But if you want them to remain quiet, you probably will have to make stretching a regular part of your life.

Here are a few suggestions to help you keep your attention on work and play, not on muscle pain:

For the neck.   To combat stiffness, hold light weights—say 3 to 5 pounds—in your hands while shrugging your shoulders. Keep your arms straight.

For the shoulders.   Place one arm, with elbow bent, behind your head, and using the opposite hand, gently pull your elbow behind your head toward your opposite shoulder. Repeat with the opposite arm.

For the wrists.   If you work on a keyboard all day, try this: Sit at a table and hold a light weight, say 3 to 5 pounds, in your hand with your palm up, your forearm supported on the table, and your wrist over the edge. Lift the weight up slowly, flexing the wrist while keeping your forearm on the table. Repeat with each wrist 10 to 20 times.

Now do the exercise as instructed above, except turn your palm toward the floor. Again use light weights and repeat 10 to 20 times.

For the knees.   Stronger muscles provide you with a stronger joint, one that's better able to withstand the considerable strain that even walking or stair-climbing places on the knees. The key is to build up quadriceps (muscles in front of the thighs) and the hamstrings (muscles in back of the legs).

Isometric knee-builder. Sit on the floor with your sore knee straight out in front of you. Place a rolled towel under the small of the knee, then tighten the muscles in your leg without moving the knee. Hold that contraction and work up to where you can keep the muscles taut for at least 30 seconds, then relax. Repeat this tightening and relaxing process up to 25 times.

Hamstring helper. Lie on your stomach with your chin to the floor. With an ankle weight (you can use a purse or a sock filled with coins and draped over the ankle) and your knee slightly bent, slowly lift the lower leg 6 to 12 inches off the floor, then slowly lower it back down, stopping before you touch the floor. Repeat the movement again, always working slowly and steadily through each repetition. Work up to doing three sets of as many of these as you comfortably can (largely determined by the amount of weight you use).

For the shins.   If you suffer shinsplints (pain and aching in the front of the leg after activity), stretching the Achilles tendon (the tendon at the back of the heel) and the calf muscles is an excellent preventive measure, says Marjorie Albohm, certified athletic trainer and associate director of the International Institute of Sports Science and Medicine at the Indiana Universty School of Medicine. "If you're a woman wearing 2-inch heels every day, you're not stretching either of those at all." Shortened calf muscles tend to throw more weight and stress forward to the shins. Stretching helps counteract the pain.

Calf stretch. Place your hands on a wall, extend one leg behind the other, and press the back heel slowly to the floor. Do this 20 times and repeat with the other leg.

For the ankles.   Sit on the floor and loop a towel around the ball of your foot while holding the ends of the towel in your hands. Alternately point your toes up and down while stretching the towel toward your face and keeping your legs straight. Repeat several times with both feet. Now toe the towel again—only this time, don't move your toes. Lean back with the towel looped around your foot until you feel the stretch in the calf muscle. Hold 15 seconds and repeat several times.

Rub Your Aches Away

Whack! You smack your funny bone. Ooww! A sudden cramp and you clench your calf. Oooh! You awake with a stiff neck. Yeeach, that shoulder is sure sore thanks to your stint as pitcher for the softball team.

What's the very first thing you do (after you let out a good yelp)? You reach out to rub where it hurts. And for good reason: rubbing works. In fact, doctors and scientists are discovering that there may be more pain-easing power in a good rub than you realize.

Experts believe that rubbing blocks the pain sensation impulses before they can reach the brain. What's more, as you continue to rub, that marvelous sensation of healing touch triggers your nervous system to release endorphins, the body's natural painkiller.

Getting a massage at different stages of an injury may even help you regain movement more quickly. In the initial inflammatory stage, when a sprained ankle is swelling, for example, massage can help drain fluid from the area, reduce swelling, and stimulate circulation. The recommended treatment is to elevate the injured area and put ice on it to counteract the heat from the inflammation. Massage is then done above the injury, stroking toward the heart.

Stroking sore muscles is also a marvelous way to combat stiffness. The long, slow, smooth massage strokes can bring fresh blood to the area and help to lengthen tissue. And the shorter "friction" strokes help break down stiffening adhesions and warm up the area around the joint, making movement easier.

Rubbing is not a cure-all.   Despite its benefits, keep in mind that rubbing can only bring you short-term relief and that it's not a substitute for proper medical care. What's more, if your pain is caused by muscle strain due to poor posture or movement habits, rubbing cannot prevent pain from recurring.

In addition, there are a few precautions to keep in mind before you lay on the hands. You should not have a rubdown if you have an infection, for instance. Avoid rubbing your legs if you have varicose veins or other blood vessel problems. A massage is okay if you have swollen limbs, but only if you rub very gently and only above the injury, and remember to stroke in the direction of your heart. Rub no closer than 6 inches on either side of bruises or broken skin.

With that said, here are guidelines for using rub power against everyday aches and pains to reduce soreness, swelling, and spasms:

Get warm before your rub.   You can get the most from a rub or massage by first warming up the affected muscles. Use a warm shower or a hydro-collator pack that you boil in water and then wrap in a towel. They send off waves of moist heat and are especially good for back problems.

Use heat-penetrating liniments with care.   Those warm-but-smelly topical painkillers—Ben-Gay, Icy Hot, Tiger Balm, and oil of wintergreen—stimulate the circulation of blood to the affected area, bringing relief. But use caution when applying them. Never use a heating pad after any of these rubs and never cover the area afterward with anything other than normal clothing. Covering or heating the liniments could increase the absorption and cause serious injury to the skin.

A better idea is to try aspirin-based creams. They're greaseless and less likely to irritate your skin, and you won't feel the heat sensation as you would with a lot of other rubs. They work like aspirin, reducing pain and inflammation.

Ice it.   While heat can prepare the body for rubbing, cooling the painful area with ice while you massage can enhance the benefits. "The intense stimulation that ice provides is an excellent way to 'close the gate' at the spinal pathway and inhibit painful information from reaching your brain," says Ronald Melzack, Ph.D., past president of the International Association for the Study of Pain and originator of the gate control theory of pain. The basic technique (for ice massage) is to slowly rub the ice in circles on the spot that hurts. Continue for 5 to 7 minutes or until the area feels numb.

Different strokes for different folks.   Certain special strokes can be employed for overuse injuries. Try out these strokes, remembering to work muscles around the area, never the bone.

Compressing the muscle. Your aim is to spread the muscle fiber and increase circulation. You simply press the belly (the wide central part) of the muscle. This stroke can be done on nearly any muscle both before and after a workout.

To relieve shin pain, for example, press on the muscle just outside the shin bone with the palm of your hand. Don't press on the shinbone itself, but work each area of the muscle belly from just below the knee to just above the ankle.

Trigger point or direct pressure. Find an area that is really tight or tender. Then press down on that point with your finger, thumb, or knuckle. Often after a few seconds the pain will release and you'll feel the tissue soften. Trigger points are often easy to find where the gluteal medius (buttock) muscles and hamstring muscles meet. When you locate this sensitive point, press with your thumb, hold for a count of five, then release.

Cross-fiber friction. This stroke is applied perpendicularly to the direction of the muscle fibers. In the top of the leg, for example, muscle fibers of the quadriceps basically run from the hip to the knee. So you should massage your leg sideways across the grain. Do this stroke so the fiber moves with the skin. Do it on tight tissue near the ends of the muscle—near either the hip or the knee.

Break Hurtful Habits

The best way to treat sore muscles is not to get them in the first place. So here's how to prevent most, if not all, muscle pain associated with exercise or bad habits.

Always warm up and stretch.   A good warm-up, one that lasts at least 10 minutes, helps prevent injuries. Warming up makes your muscles more elastic—easier to stretch and thus harder to injure. The best preparation for exercise is to take a brisk walk, ride a stationary bike, do push-ups or sit-ups or any activity that will make you break into a light sweat. You can even take a warm bath or shower.

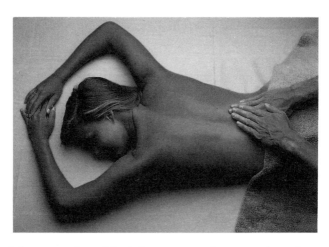

A rubdown can be a blissful way to soothe muscular aches, increase blood flow, and prevent stiffness. For the best benefits, warm up the affected area with moist heat. Gently move skin over underlying tissue (don't rub the bone) and massage in the direction of the heart. Stop if the pain increases. Don't rub a serious injury or an inflamed area.

Follow your warm-up by going through gentle stretches or range-of-motion exercises for each limb. Simply stretch your arms and legs to the point of tightness and then extend a wee bit further. Hold for a few seconds, release, and repeat. Never bounce.

Taper off your exercise workout.   After hard exercise or physical work, the bloodstream is loaded with lactic acid, which collects in the bloodstream when there is a lack of oxygen, explains Gabe Mirkin, M.D., of the Sportsmedicine Institute in Silver Spring, Maryland, author of *Dr. Gabe Mirkin's Fitness Clinic.* When the acid reaches high levels, it disrupts normal chemical reactions of the muscles and can make your muscles hurt. "The most effective way to clear the bloodstream is to continue exercising at a slow, relaxed pace," Dr. Mirkin advises.

Cool down by reducing the pace of your activity, then stretch as you did before your activity.

Drink up.   The typical muscle cramp is a heat cramp,

caused by dehydration from profuse sweating. After all, a hard exercise can make you lose 4 to 6 pounds of water in an hour. Something's got to give. So your muscles give you cramps. To counteract cramping, drink water before, during, and after physical activity.

Make sure your shoe fits the activity.   The main risk from trying to make one shoe do everything is injury. Consider that running shoes chiefly cushion the foot, but are unstable for a side-to-side activity like tennis or other court games. On the other hand, racquet shoes have very little shock absorption but brace and stablize the foot so you don't turn your ankle. What this means is that if you play tennis wearing a running shoe, you could almost literally fall off your shoes, because they are not designed to handle that kind of side-to-side motion. Note: workout and aerobic shoes are designed to absorb shock *and* stabilize your foot.

If you participate in activities that cause a lot of forefoot impact, judge a shoe on its ability to absorb shock in that area. The best test is to try the shoes on in the store and jump up and down, both on the toes and flat-footed. The impact with the floor should be firm but not jarring.

Update your shoes.   "If your shoes can't take the shock any more," says Gary M. Gordon, D.P.M., of the University of Pennsylvania Sports Medicine Center in Philadelphia, "well, that shock has to go someplace."

Where it goes is through your foot, up your shin, and into the knee. Sometimes it keeps on going, up to the hip and back as well.

"I tell runners that if they run 25 miles a week or more, they need new shoes every two or three months," Dr. Gordon says. "If they run less than that, they need new shoes every four to six months. Aerobic dancers, basketball and tennis players who work out twice a week can probably get by on new shoes every four to six months. If they're doing it up to four times or more a week, they also need new shoes every two months."

Change to a softer running surface.   If you participate in aerobic dance, be aware that injuries are highest on concrete floors covered with carpet, while wood floors over airspace are the least damaging. If you must dance on a nonresilient floor, make sure the instructor teaches only low-impact aerobics or that high-quality foam mats are provided. If you are a runner, choose grass or dirt over asphalt, and choose asphalt over concrete. Concrete is very unyielding and should be avoided as much as possible.

Get into low gear.   Biking—either stationary or free-wheel—is a great way to stay in shape and take a load off your knees if you do it with caution. Cyclists can damage their knees, typically by thinking that the harder it is to pedal, the more exercise they get.

So, depending on the type of biking you do (steep hills are not advised), riding may still be too strenuous. Fast pedaling in gears that feel easy is what you want. In general, a lower gear (easier to pedal) is a better gear for your muscles and joints.

Never play through the pain.   If you only feel the pain of tendinitis (soreness and inflammation around a joint) during or after exercise, and if it isn't too bad, you may be thinking that you could run a race or swim laps with that same amount of pain—if you had to. Or maybe you already have.

In either case, you would be wise to realign your thinking. You shouldn't play through pain unless your physician or physical therapist tells you otherwise, experts say. If pain is severe and you continue to abuse the tendon, it may rupture. And that could mean a long layoff, surgery, or even permanent disability.

"The most important thing to understand is that if an exercise causes increasing discomfort or pain, then stop," says James M. Fox, M.D., director of the Center for Disorders of the Knee in Van Nuys, California. "You have to listen to your body and not simply assume that you need to 'work through the pain.' God gave you pain for a reason."

Keep your wrists straight.   As mentioned before, carpal tunnel syndrome results when pressure is constantly applied to the median nerve when the wrist is flexed up or down. Some workers are affected more than others, especially meat cutters, cashiers, data processors, assembly line workers, truck drivers—the kind of people who absolutely must use their hands on the job. Those who work at home are at risk, too. Carpal tunnel syndrome has been known to attack homemakers who spend lots of time wringing wet laundry by hand, sweeping with a broom, dicing with a knife, or even shelling peas. Even do-it-yourself weekend carpenters can do themselves in. Excessive use of a staple gun over a weekend is enough to trigger the disease, for instance.

"If the wrist is repeatedly flexed and extended, the pressure is increased. To avoid this, keep your hands and wrists as straight as possible while typing, driving, or working around the house," advises John Sebright, M.D., a Michigan plastic surgeon who limits his practice to surgery of the hand. Here are a few more wrist-saving suggestions.

- Handle tools with care. Don't concentrate pressure at the base of the wrist when using hand tools. Use your elbow and shoulder as much as possible.

- Adjust your keyboard. If you have long hands and fingers, you can reduce the strain by adjusting the keyboard to a more horizontal position (flat with the work surface) as long as it does not put your arms or shoulders in a strained position. For those who have short hands and fingers, a higher incline on the keyboard, typewriter, or calculator will make the keys easier to reach.

- Use the right grip. If you have to carry anything with a handle, be sure the grip fits your hand. If the grip is too small, build it up with tape or rubberized tubing. If it's too large, get another handle.

Best Balms for Aching Feet

Along with "Hello," "Goodbye," "How are you?," and "I didn't do it," one of the most often repeated phrases in any language has to be "My feet are killing me."

No wonder. The human foot is a complex mechanism, with more bones than a $10 bucket of fried chicken and an intricate network of muscles, ligaments, nerves, and blood vessels. Most of us have little understanding of what makes our feet work, much less how to prevent problems. Add that to the fact that more of us are walking, jogging, and running our way to better health but neglecting our feet until something goes wrong, and it's easy to see why foot ailments are among the most common health problems in the country.

"If people gave half as much thought to foot health as they did to foot fashion, we could prevent a lot of problems," says Norman Klombers, D.P.M., executive director of the American Podiatric Medical Association.

Practically all of us are born with healthy feet. But by the time we become adults, 70 percent of us develop foot problems. Heredity, improper foot care (including that caused by shoes, socks, or stockings that don't fit properly), injury, and the loss of muscle and ligament tone that comes with aging are among the most common causes of problems. Women suffer four times as many foot ailments as men, with high-heeled shoes often to blame.

Your feet carry a heavy load and need all the consideration they can get. If you're like most people, you walk several miles daily, usually on hard, unyielding surfaces, and about 115,000 miles in a lifetime—more than four times around the earth. The feet of most active people absorb the impact of up to five million pounds a day. That's a lot of pounding, and where there's pounding, there's usually pain.

Fortunately, where there's pain, you'll generally find a way to conquer it. Here are some self-help hints to help you fight foot pain.

Relieving the Agony of De Feet

Feet are dermatological wonders. The skin on your soles is up to ten times thicker than elsewhere on your body, for protection and padding. Unfortunately, the rest of your feet are covered with ordinary, easily damaged skin, which is why skin-related problems are the main reason people visit podiatrists.

But most skin-related foot problems are easy to treat and even easier to prevent. Here's how to treat some of the more common problems:

Blisters.   Excessive friction and pressure on the skin are a main cause of blisters. If you can get to your blister easily and it's not too severe, you can handle it yourself. If there are signs of blood inside the blister or if it becomes infected, see your podiatrist.

To drain a small blister, sterilize a sewing needle with 70 percent isopropyl alcohol. Clean the blistered skin with an antiseptic and make small holes to release the fluid. Blot the fluid with a piece of sterile gauze. An antibiotic cream may be applied and covered with a protective pad.

To prevent blisters, you can apply moleskin padding to areas that, because of the shape of your foot, may rub against every pair of shoes you own, constantly causing the sores. (Moleskin is available at most drugstores.)

Skin that's too dry or too sweaty is also prone to blisters. Apply a thin coat of petroleum jelly to dry skin before activity. If your feet sweat a lot, cornstarch sprinkled in shoes and socks helps.

Corns.   Those small, circular, hard areas of skin cells, typically found on top of a toe joint or on the sole of the foot, are one of the most common foot afflictions.

Because corns are usually caused by shoe friction against a contracted toe, the easiest way to avoid them is to wear only properly fitting footwear. If your shoes don't rub against your toes, it's doubtful you'll ever develop a corn. Soft corns can develop between toes if shoes are too narrow.

If you have a corn, don't try to cut it off with a razor blade. Bathroom surgery can lead to infections, says Marc A. Brenner, D.P.M., of Glendale, New York, past president of the American Society of Podiatric Dermatology. "A doctor using sterilized instruments can do this safely and with little pain, but it's dangerous for anyone to try it at home."

He also advises against the home remedy of soaking your feet and then using sandpaper or a callus file to grind away the corn. "You can cause a more serious problem, such as an infection, and not correct the cause of the corn. Even if it works, the corn will probably reappear in three to five weeks."

Over-the-counter corn-removal medications should be avoided because they contain an acid that penetrates the hard skin surface but can burn the surrounding soft, healthy skin. Podiatrists treat many skin ulcers caused by these products.

To ease the pain of a corn until you can get to a doctor, try soaking your feet in a pan of warm water with about a cup of Epsom salts. You can also pour in ½ cup of white vinegar to take the sting and soreness out. Put some moleskin around the corn.

If you wear wide-toed shoes but still suffer from corns, the cause may be a biomechanical fault, such as a hammertoe, in which the knuckle of the toe rises above its normal position and rubs the top of the shoe because of the poor mechanics of the foot. Another cause can be an underlying bone spur, a bony growth created when local inflammation is present over an extended period of time. X-rays may be needed to determine the problem and necessary treatment if the cause is biomechanical.

Calluses.   These hard, thickened clumps usually appear on the heel or ball of the foot and can be treated in the same way as you treat corns.

Mild calluses can usually be handled at home. But be patient. Attacking callused skin too aggressively can irritate it and do more harm than good. Use a pumice stone or Buf-Puf to remove a few layers of callused skin each night. Never use a razor blade on calluses because of the risk of infection.

Calluses are difficult to prevent because they are not caused by your shoes but by your foot structure and the way you walk.

"Insoles are often prescribed to reduce the friction that causes calluses," says Dr. Brenner. Orthoses, or custom shoe inserts, are designed to accommodate your calluses if the cause is an out-of-line bone that hits the ground harder than other foot bones. Orthoses also help restore foot balance. With chronic calluses, surgery may be necessary to correct an underlying structural problem.

Infection Protection

The warm, moist, dark environment inside your shoes makes a perfect breeding ground for viruses, bacteria, and fungi. With a little care, you can stamp out these foot infections. Here's how.

Stay fungus-free.   The area between your toes is prone to skin problems, and the most common is a contagious fungal infection known as *athlete's foot.* The best way to keep the fungi out of your loafers is to create an inhospitable environment by wearing shoes made of natural materials, such as leather and canvas, that let moisture escape and feet breathe. Dust inside the shoes with cornstarch before and after wearing to absorb moisture. Keep your shoes dry and try not to wear them on consecutive days because it takes a day or two for them to dry completely.

Bathe your feet at least once a day using soap and water, and be sure to dry thoroughly between your toes. It helps to change your socks twice a day, and if your feet sweat excessively, wear socks made of cotton or some "wicking" fiber, because they keep feet cooler and drier.

Another way to prevent the flaking, cracking, itching, burning skin caused by fungal infections is to apply an over-the-counter medicated powder to your shoes each day. If the problem persists, a podiatrist can prescribe a stronger medication.

It also helps to wear thongs or other protective footwear wherever a fungus may be lurking, such as around the community pool or in the showers at the local health club.

Ward off warts.   The same precautionary footwear can shield your feet against the virus that causes *plantar warts,* painful skin growths that occur on the soles of the feet. They are caused by a highly contagious virus that can be contracted by stepping on a wet, abrasive, virus-infected surface. Abrasion helps rub the virus into the skin on the bottom of your foot, which explains why they generally occur on weight-bearing areas.

The virus thrives in the same warm, moist conditions that help foster the athlete's foot fungus, so preventive measures are the same for both.

A wart should never be handled with an over-the-counter medication. "Check with a podiatrist to make sure you have a wart, and not a callus, corn, or skin cancer," says Dr. Brenner. A podiatrist has a wide array of treatment alternatives that may include dry ice, vitamin A injections, acid treatments, surgically scooping out the wart, or vaporizing it with a laser. But be aware that regardless of the method used, there's a 5 to 15 percent chance that the wart will grow back.

Plantar warts are slow growing. If you spot a suspicious growth on your foot, have it checked immediately because a wart is easier to treat when small. More important, warts can spread to other parts of your foot, hands, and even other areas of skin if not checked.

When an itch means allergy.   If you notice that the skin on your feet is irritated, itchy, red, and painful, with small blisters, you may conclude that you have athlete's foot. But it could be contact dermatitis, an allergic skin reaction to some substance, perhaps nail polish, soap, foot powder, spray, or shoe material. Contact dermatitis is often mistaken for a fungal or bacterial infection.

To both treat and prevent the condition, find out what you're allergic to and avoid it. If the problem can't be traced to a medication, food, or cosmetic product, special hypoallergenic shoes may be needed. Avoid using strong soaps and detergents and instead use gentle, hypoallergenic products to cleanse the skin. Over-the-counter preparations containing cortisone may help, but see a podiatrist if your condition fails to respond to the medication.

Foot Problems You Were Born With

A few common foot ailments have little to do with lack of consideration for your feet and are instead the result of inborn problems. Your podiatrist and the treatments below may be the best course of relief for the following conditions.

Bunions.   Despite popular belief, bunions are usually hereditary and aren't caused by improperly fitted shoes, although pointed shoes aggravate and accelerate bunion formation.

A bunion starts as a small enlargement on the side of the big toe and grows over the years. Because it's the result of faulty foot structure and function, there are no self-care measures or ways to prevent the condition. "Surgery is the only way to correct the bone problem," says John McCrea, D.P.M., of Beloit, Wisconsin, "and then orthoses may be necessary to control any abnormal motion. If we can spot potential bunion problems in young patients, we can design orthoses that may help prevent future problems."

Flat feet.   An inborn structural or functional defect is also often the cause of flat feet. Totally flat, archless feet are rare, however, and most people who think they have the condition actually have normally low arches. Low or flat arches won't keep you out of the army anymore, but they can cause a strain that may lead to discomfort in the foot, knee, hip, or lower back.

"Collapsed arches are quite common in people in their fifties and sixties. When the arch starts to give way, orthoses can be used for support. This should prevent the strained ligaments that lead to other problems,'' Dr. McCrea says.

High arches.   This structural formation can also cause discomfort because the ball of the foot and heel absorb the total impact while walking. Shoes with good shock-absorbing qualities are crucial, and orthoses may be needed for extra support.

Gout.   Yet another inborn condition that can lead to foot problems is how your body deals with uric acid. The inner workings of some people either produce too much uric acid or can't remove what's created. The result is a metabolic disease called gout, in which crystals of the uric acid accumulate in body joints, often the big-toe joint.

Gout attacks are sudden and very painful, and even the weight of a bed sheet on a swollen, gouty toe can be agonizing. The condition, a form of arthritis, is most prevalent in middle-aged men and is often seen in families.

In some susceptible people, foods high in substances known as purines, such as sardines, shellfish, anchovies, liver, sweetbreads, and the like, can trigger a uric-acid increase and a gout attack, as can alcohol and some medications.

Besides suggesting dietary changes, a podiatrist may prescribe an anti-inflammatory medication or one that controls uric-acid levels. In rare cases, repeated attacks can leave a toe stiff, and surgery or orthotics may be required.

Nails You Shouldn't Pound

Your toenails are protective devices that occasionally cause discomfort if not properly cared for.

Ingrown toenails.   This is the most common and painful nail condition, occurring when the side of the nail digs into the skin. Improper nail cutting is generally the cause, although a toe injury or fungal infection can also trigger problems.

Ingrown toenails can be easily avoided by using good, clean clippers designed to cut the nail straight across—not rounded to match the shape of the toe and not too short. Many ingrown nails result from picking or ripping the nails, which usually leaves a small piece, known as a spicule, to easily grow into the skin. Cutting into the corners of your nails can also lead to spicule formation.

To help relieve some of the discomfort until you can get to a podiatrist, soak your foot in lukewarm water to soften the nail, then tuck a small wisp of cotton between the offending nail edge and the skin. "This provides temporary relief but does nothing to cure the problem," says Dr. Brenner. "It also doesn't do any good to cut a V in the center of the nail. The nail won't grow toward the center and away from the ingrown edge, as some people believe. All nails grow from back to front only."

Over-the-counter remedies that contain tannic acid may help toughen the skin on the side of the nail and resist ingrowing in some cases. Avoid those that contain other kinds of acids, because they often are too harsh.

Injured toenails.   Drop something on your feet, and before you know it, your toenails will turn black and blue, and the pressure from blood collecting under the nail will produce a whopping pain. While there are several home remedies that have been around for years, consult a podiatrist, who'll use an electronic needle or drill to safely relieve the pressure.

Your toenails can also turn black and blue if they stub against your shoe during activity, in which case either the nails are too long or, more likely, your shoes don't fit.

Special Treats for Tired Feet

Few of us think about our feet at all until they hurt. The rest of the time, we simply use them as if there's no tomorrow.

So what can you do at the end of a long, hard day when your feet cry uncle? Here are five ways to pamper your tired tootsies:

Put your feet up.   Elevate your feet at a 45-degree angle to your body and relax for 20 minutes. Raising your feet will get your circulation going.

Try a foot soak.   A tried-and-true foot revitalizer is to soak your feet in a basin of warm water containing 1 or 2 tablespoons of Epsom salts, says Maryland podiatrist Mark Sussman, D.P.M. Rinse with clear, cool water, then pat your feet dry and massage in a moisturizing gel or cream.

Run hot and cold.   Dr. Sussman recommends a treatment popular at European spas. Sit on the edge of the bathtub and hold your feet under running water for several minutes (alternate 1 minute of comfortably hot water with 1 minute of cold, ending with the cold). The contrasting baths will invigorate your whole system. If you have a shower massage attachment, use it for

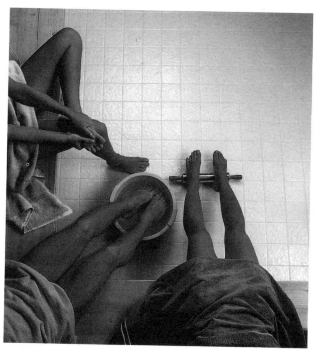

Here's a pain-relieving trio for tired feet. Start with a warm water and Epsom salt soak. Next, apply oil and use your thumbs to gently stroke your foot, starting at the heel. Move on to the arch, then gently caress the ball of the foot. Advance to the toes, softly pulling and stroking each. Finally, glide your feet over a rolling pin to build up aching arch muscles.

Shoe Savvy

Don't ruin all your foot-care efforts by wearing the wrong shoes. If a certain pair of shoes hurts your feet, experts suggest you give them the boot. Poorly fitting shoes can actually change the shape of your toes.

Here are some shoe buying—and wearing—hints for healthier feet.

- **Shop in the afternoon.** Your feet swell a bit during the day. Get shoes that are comfortable, not ones you have to break in. And always try them on, since manufacturers' sizes differ.
- **Fit the larger foot.** Have your feet measured while standing, and since almost everyone has one foot that's bigger than the other, fit the larger one.
- **Roomy is best.** The shoe should be roomy enough to allow a thumb's width between the end of the big toe and the tip of the shoe but not so loose that your foot slides around. The widest part of your foot should correspond to the widest part of the shoe. Never buy a shoe that's not comfortable in the store on the theory that it will stretch out as you wear it. And never buy shoes if you can see the side of the shoe is stretched out by your foot.
- **Go for thick soles.** Try wearing shoes with thick, shock-absorbing soles to shield your feet from rough surfaces and hard pavements. Don't let

an even more stimulating workout. But as always, if you have diabetes or impaired circulation, don't expose your feet to extremes of temperature.

Cool off your hot dogs.   Another way to refresh tired feet is to wrap a few ice cubes in a wet washcloth, then rub it over your feet and ankles for a few minutes. Ice acts to relieve any inflammation, says Bethlehem, Pennsylvania, podiatrist Neal Kramer, D.P.M., and it also serves as a mild anesthetic. Then dry your feet your soles become too thin or worn, because they just won't do the job they're supposed to.

- **Invest in insoles.** High heels cause your foot to pitch forward as you walk, putting painful pressure on the ball of your foot. To prevent this discomfort, wear a half-insole to help keep your foot in place. And be sure to take the insoles with you to the shoe store to ensure that they'll fit comfortably in your new shoes.

- **Stretch your shoes.** When you add insoles to shoes you already have, make sure they don't cramp your toes. If things are tight, you may be able to stretch the shoes to accommodate the insoles. Fill a sock with sand, stuff it into the shoe's toe box, and wrap the shoe with a wet towel. Let it dry out over the next 24 hours. Repeat once or twice if needed.

- **Change heel heights.** Women's thin-soled, pointy-toed high heels are classic villains in foot pain. Wearing high heels tightens the calf muscles, which leads to foot fatigue, says John Waller, Jr., M.D., an orthopedic surgeon from New York. If you must dress up for work, ease foot strain by wearing walking or athletic shoes to and from the job and switching to heels at the office.

and swab them with witch hazel, cologne, alcohol, or vinegar for a cooling and drying effect.

Massage away your aches.   Either before or during a soak, give yourself a nice little foot massage. Work over the whole foot, squeezing the toes gently, then pressing in a circular motion over the bottom of your foot. One really effective movement is to slide your thumb as hard as you can in the arch of the foot.

Exercise Away Foot Fatigue

Many doctors recommend that you exercise your feet and leg muscles throughout the day to ward off aches and keep the circulation going. Try these exercises first chance you get:

- If your feet feel tense and cramped any time during the day, give them a good shake, as you would your hands if they felt cramped. Do one foot at a time, then relax and flex your toes up and down.

- If you must stand for long periods of time, walk in place whenever you can. Keep changing your stance and try to rest one foot on a stool or step occasionally. If possible, stand on carpeting or a spongy rubber mat.

- To relieve stiffness, remove your shoes, sit in a chair, and stretch your feet out in front of you. Circle both feet from the ankles ten times in one direction, then ten times in the other. Point toes down as far as possible, then flex them up as high as you can. Repeat ten times. Now grasp your toes and gently pull them back and forth.

- To relieve strain on the arches, rest your weight on the outer borders of your feet, then roll them inward.

- To ease tightness in your ankles and arches, stand flat on your feet, rise to your toes, and repeat several times.

- Strengthen toes and muscles on top of the foot by sitting in a relaxed position with your bare feet on the floor. Try to pick up a towel, a pencil, or marbles with your toes.

- For a nice mini-massage, remove your shoes and roll each foot over a golf ball, tennis ball, or rolling pin for a minute or two.

- Or put a handful of dried beans in moccasin-style slippers, slip them on, and walk around the room several times—you'll get a massage-like workout on the soles of your feet.